EAT LIKE AN ELEPHANT
LOOK LIKE AN ANGEL

TRANSFORM YOUR BELIEFS, LOVE YOUR BODY
AND LOSE WEIGHT EATING ANYTHING YOU WANT!

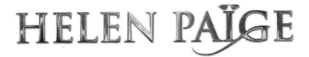

Eat Like an Elephant
Look Like an Angel

Transform your beliefs, love your body and lose weight eating anything you want!

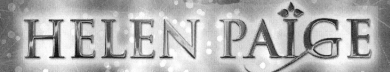

HELEN PAIGE

Eat Like An Elephant Look Like An Angel
By Helen Paige
www.HelenPaige.com

Published by Angelos Publishing
Text copyright © Helen Paige 2016

Cover design by Laura Gordon.

National Library of Australia Cataloguing-in-Publication entry.

Creator:	Paige, Helen- author.
Title:	Eat like an elephant look like an angel : transform your beliefs, love your body and lose weight eating anything you want! / Helen Paige.
Edition:	2nd edition.
ISBN:	9780980554229 (paperback)
Notes:	Includes bibliographical references.
Subjects:	Weight loss--Psychological aspects. Food--Psychological aspects.

DISCLAIMER

This book contains the opinions and ideas of its author. It is intended to provide helpful and informative material on the subjects addressed in the publication; it is not intended to diagnose, prescribe, or treat any health disorder or other serious personal issue, nor is it guaranteeing any particular results. This book is sold with the understanding that the author and publisher are not engaged in rendering medical, health or any other kind of personal professional services in the book, and the reader should consult with such person(s) before adopting any of the suggestions in this book or drawing inferences from it. The author and publisher specifically disclaim all responsibility for any liability, loss or risk, personal or otherwise, which is incurred as a consequence, directly or indirectly, of the use and application of any of the contents of this book.

ABOUT THIS BOOK

This book is not going to teach you what to eat or what not to eat in order to lose weight. If you are reading this, chances are you are already an expert on what you consider good food and bad. Instead, this book is about making food meaningless to you, in the sense that it will never again matter what you eat or what you do not eat. Food will cease to make you fat, and food will cease to make you thin. You will understand and create the reality where food ceases to have any impact on your body. You will be guided to create a body consciousness where you no longer react to food as you have in the past.

The intent of this book is to change the very fabric of your mental and physical consciousness, so you move from a place of being a victim to food to a place of true self-actualization. You will be guided to reach a level of mind and body consciousness that is mastery, enlightenment, knowing and being. From this place within yourself you will no longer need to control your life or body, but will instead trust life and trust your body. You will cease to be a victim to food. You will stop reacting to life and instead harness a great creative energy and live from this place each and every day. You will go from a place of being reactive to food and reactive to life to a place of being able to create whatever you desire. Do you wish to create a healthier, leaner body? Easy! Do you want to be able to eat anything you want? Effortless!

You are about to embark on an amazing new journey. A journey like never before. It is time, if you are truly ready, to change the way you view food, forever. Now is the time to transform the effects of food on your body and on your life.

CONTENTS

HELEN PAIGE

INTRODUCTION

I have called this book *Eat Like an Elephant Look Like an Angel* for a very distinct reason. Funnily enough it has nothing to do with elephants eating a lot and angels being thin. Rather elephants represent an overcoming of obstacles, and for many, being in a physical body is the greatest obstacle of all. Many people feel limited by the constraints of the physical because it appears to have so many boundaries. You have been led to believe that if you do not follow its rules, it rebels or decays on you. I do not believe this is true. I believe that you chose this body and as you learn to live within it, you will learn to teach and guide it well. It abides by your rules, by your laws, and not the other way around.

As you progress past the "elephant" obstacles of your thinking you will discover the amazing "angel" ability that you have to create from a place of love and peace. This is the journey of elephants and angels—to be able to overcome your previous obstacles that turn food into fat, and instead turn food into pure energy that is effortlessly released from your body.

I wrote this book initially for myself because I wanted another way of being when it comes to my body, my weight, and my relationship with food. I spent many of my younger years doing weight control in all sorts of crazy ways: overexercising, purging, starving, and dieting. At the time these often-extreme measures made sense to me. I exercised, ate well, and still gained weight if I followed the healthy food guidelines specifying how much to eat in a day. I feared weight gain more than anything else in the world and believed that being thin meant being happy. Emotionally at that time, I was also in a great deal of inner turmoil and the only way I knew to live my life was through extreme control of both myself and my environment. A perfectionist, I always needed to reflect on the outside what society expected of me, or perhaps truer to the word, what I expected of myself.

Over the years I was lucky enough to embark on an inner healing journey where I no longer battled with food in the same way, but I was still left with an extreme set of rules about what I could and couldn't eat in order to remain thin. After years of such extreme self-control, I remember vividly one year at Christmas being fed up watching everyone else enjoying their food, except for me. Instead I was busy thinking of what food I wouldn't be allowed to eat next week to make up for what

I was eating that day. Something in me snapped! It was as if a part of me said, *'I've had enough! From this day forward I want to eat too!'* Not that I hadn't been eating, but my day consisted of eating what I considered "safe" food, while thinking about food all day long and not allowing myself to eat what I genuinely desired.

So I embarked on this quest, this journey, of exploring a different way of eating. It was a quest to find a different way of relating to food and a different way of relating to my body. This journey led me through the frontiers of mind/body medicine where others claimed they had found a way to change the body so that it no longer reacted to food and no longer gained weight. In other words, the claim was that I would be able to eat whatever I wanted and my body would just eliminate the excess, ensuring I wouldn't gain weight. My excitement at discovering such approaches was intermingled with fear of failure as I tried these methods of eating and failed. Still, something in me knew this way of eating was a potential reality for me. I knew it was possible. I just didn't know how to create it in myself yet.

Determined to succeed where other approaches appeared to fail me, I drew on my years of incidental research through over fifteen years of working seeming miracles with clients, helping them overcome what appeared as incurable health conditions. Working as a medical intuitive over this time, I had assisted countless people to correct the true cause of their weight gain. What I learned was that people's weight gain and failure to lose weight was rarely to do with the food they were eating and more often about unresolved emotions, limiting beliefs, low self-esteem, and a depleted energy system. As a medical intuitive I have the ability to "see" what is occurring in the body and within the energy system. I can perceive where physical distress and life issues originate. Using this information I can assist in erasing old causative factors, and guide the client to transform their thinking, their body, and ultimately their health.

The more I read and researched, the more I found evidence, much of it from science, that proved the body was more a result of thinking, rather than genes, bad luck, and the food ingested. The role of one's emotional health, belief systems, and thoughts began to rise to the surface as the key to change and permanent transformation. If others had done it, I knew I could too.

Excited to be allowed finally to love my body and to love food and know that they are not both against me, I now offer this information to you.

This book consists of two parts. Part 1 will provide you with the blueprint to change the way you relate to food and the way food relates to you. It will show you the way to break free from food as being the cause of weight change and will empower you with the tools to be able to eat anything you like without effect.

Following on from this, Part 2 consists of eighty-one days of my journey as I have directly journaled my own inner changes and understandings along the way. The purpose of this eighty-one-day period is to begin the process of discovering and changing your own deep beliefs and thought patterns that up until now have been turning what you eat into excess energy. I encourage you, as you read my record of eighty-one days, to journal your own insights and inspirations, recording your own eighty-one days of change. During these eighty-one days you will be cultivating a new way of being, a new way of perceiving, and a new set of beliefs that cannot be corrupted by a world convinced that food is the enemy. You are the only enemy you need to make peace with. You will also discover some life changing information through my own eighty-one-day journey that you can apply to how you relate to food and your body, so don't feel tempted to skip this part of the book.

You will notice throughout the book that most of the time I make reference to females, but I want to point out that this book is for everyone, male and female alike. So put your seat belt on, and if you are brave enough to embark on this journey, I promise, you will never regret it. The worst thing that can happen is you don't lose any weight and this approach doesn't work for you. Oh well, at least you tried. But what is the best thing that can possibly happen? Perhaps being able to eat whatever you want and never gain weight again, and better still lose or gain weight as you want to. Are you excited, and a little bit frightened? I was too. I promise it's worth a try. Now cross your fingers, count to ten and . . . here we go!

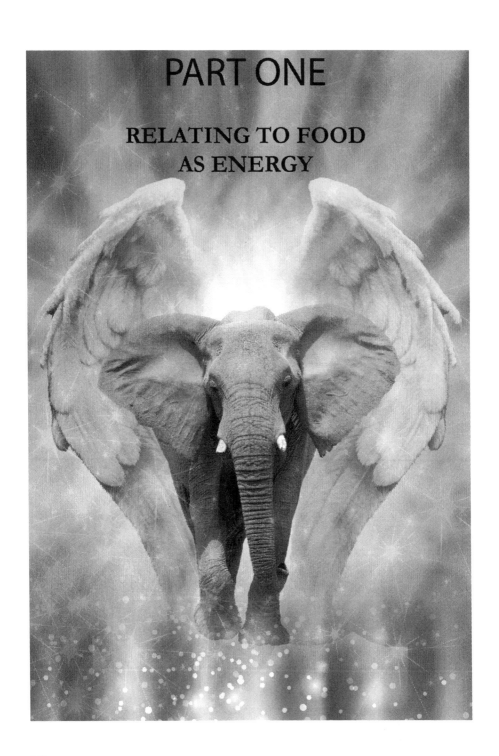

PART ONE

RELATING TO FOOD
AS ENERGY

CHAPTER 1
CONVINCE ME THIS WORKS!

As I see it, I am proposing what many people will consider a preposterous notion! I am proposing to you that you can eat ANYTHING, and I mean any food at all, and as much as you like, and still lose weight. Every weight-loss system, no matter how sophisticated, still has as its underlying foundation the assumption that, in order to lose weight, you need to eat less and move more. I am suggesting that weight loss has little to do with this and instead everything to do with how you think, how you feel, and what you believe to be true for you.

You have probably tried many of the diets or eating approaches available on the market today. You may be one of the many who are caught up in the weight-loss industry's merry-go-round. This merry-go-round approach includes undertaking diet after diet, struggling to either lose weight or keep it off, and endlessly searching for some perfect approach to both exercise and eating so that you can stay slim forever. So many people caught up in these cycles of thinking and action seem to view the body as never being quite good enough. Whatever their fad way of eating today, they will be easily swayed tomorrow by the latest and greatest way to lose weight. In this way of thinking, you never stop looking for a way to lose weight and you are always perceiving yourself as a problem to be solved.

You would think that with so many weight-loss approaches on the market today there is no reason for anyone to be overweight, and yet as a collective we are fatter today than we have ever been. I am amazed that even the skinniest of women, who appear to have it all together, still reach out and buy the latest magazine that promises weight loss, or the latest weight-loss book. I am, in effect, hoping this is the last weight-loss book you ever buy. I am hoping that this book encourages you to see your inner value and to be set free from the effects of food once and for all. Gregg Braden in *The Divine Matrix* points out that quantum research has shown that: "The consciousness of the observer determines how energy will behave" and that "The focus of our awareness becomes the reality of our world." In other words, how you think and feel determines the outcomes of your body and your life. In order to create change in your life, you need to feel the change you want as though it is here for you now. This is the possibility presented to you through this book.

I could perhaps attempt to convince you to get off the dieting merry-go-round by presenting you with research statistics that indicate that 95 percent of people who lose weight eventually gain it back within three years and that, beyond three years, the failure rate is even worse. While this may be true, I prefer to have you CHOOSE this approach because the only research statistic you need to convince you is YOU—your life so far with food. You are the only statistic that matters to me, and the only one that need matter to you. How many times have you failed to look and feel the weight you want to be? How often are you trying to control your weight through dieting or food restrictions? How often do you obsessively think about eating? You are the only statistic that matters. You are the reason to dedicate yourself to this approach so you can finally be free of your issues around food.

You are being offered the opportunity to be able to eat anything and never again gain weight. You are being offered a chance to be able to eat anything you like and still lose weight. No more avoiding certain foods, obsessively counting calories, or getting tempted to eat what the experts say you should be eating. No more thinking about food. Instead you can release all this compulsiveness and begin eating with pleasure and joy, and begin truly loving yourself. You can eat without guilt, without worry, and without fear. You can just eat.

I am asking you to convince yourself this is right for you, because it *feels* right and because you have been drawn to the truth of what I write from my own deep intuitive levels to your deep intuitive levels. You do not really need to be convinced at all. All you need is just a bit of faith and the rest will convince you along the way!

In her book *Body Image: Understanding Body Dissatisfaction in Men, Women and Children*, Sarah Grogan points out some poignant and surprising findings based on the latest research, including: the diet industry promotes a very thin ideal of the body to strive for; health problems due to dieting are likely and rarely lead to long-term weight loss; being slightly overweight may even have beneficial effects on women; body dissatisfaction is what leads many people to diet rather than a genuine weight issue; in Western societies slimness is associated with success and happiness; a public that "feels fat" is an easy target for the dieting industry; and what we consider to be the slim ideal for both men and women is largely dependent on cultural factors rather than health. This is a book worth reading. These are eye-opening suggestions that research has uncovered and much can be expanded upon each item mentioned, but I raise them here to allow you to see that there is so much more to the whole weight-loss issue than simply losing weight. Perhaps our obsession with weight loss in the first place is the thing that needs to change.

STAGES OF BODY CONSCIOUSNESS

I have developed the following four stages of body consciousness through the many years of working with people who want to lose weight. They are developmental stages of thinking, detailing the levels of how you relate to your body, your weight, and to food. You may even find yourself relating to several of these stages at once. This is normal. This is the starting point for you to identify your current perceptions. Use these various stages and the information within them as a guide only. The important thing is to gain awareness through them, rather than self-judgment from them. Along the way in life, the most important quality and attitude you can adopt toward yourself is one of self-forgiveness. It is only through forgiving your every thought, action, and behavior that you will move on to bigger and better things. People who get caught in cycles of self-judgment can stay there for a very long time. Instead you can choose the easy path through self-forgiveness. I cannot choose it for you however. I can only show you the way. You need to choose it for yourself.

STAGE 1: COPYCAT

The copycat stage is all about being guided by others and wanting to be like other people in order to gain external love and approval. For most of us, this begins by unconsciously following the thinking, behavior, and deeper beliefs of our parents. For females, it is doing what you see your mother do, and for males it is often following your father's example or vice versa. I find at the workshops I have run, the first thing people say about their eating habits or perception of their body relates back to either their mother or father. Basically, you are born wanting to be like them, and if they think negatively about their own bodies, overeat, and never think they are good enough, you unconsciously copy and imitate them.

Knowing and acknowledging the beliefs and practices of your parents in relation to food, weight, and the body is important, as it allows you to observe more objectively your own habits and perceptions in light of this knowledge. How much of what you actually believe and do is based on your own unique choices and how much is based on your subconscious beliefs born in childhood?

Following on from your parents, you are also influenced and "copy" other significant people in your life, people you look up to and/or are under the care of. What you experience at school is also relevant and as you grow into a teenager; the thinking, behavior, and perceptions of your peers become your guiding light. You copy your friends in order to fit in, to gain friendships, and in order to be liked.

On the other hand sometimes the copycat stage can create rebellion in you. On a subconscious level you are attached to all that you copy, but on a conscious level you may hate this about yourself and openly rebel. This rebellion often takes the shape of putting on excessive weight to rebel against society's warped values. When this happens, however, it is the overweight rebel that suffers. It isn't really a solution for you but just another problem.

Somewhere, from when you were a baby following your inner urge to eat naturally, you lost yourself to all that you observed around you. Your thoughts, behaviors, and perceptions of yourself are no longer the real you, as you just want to fit in, gain approval, and be loved. You become the voices around you and your own inner voice is drowned out and barely heard. This is the first stage.

Some examples of the type of thinking in this stage:

- Whatever my mother/father believe, I must believe.

- I want to be like these important people in my life, therefore I need to think like they do.

- I want to be loved so I need to be like them and do as they do.

- If the important adults and role models do this, then it must be right.

- The external world is my guide.

- I am unconsciously following the lead of the important people in my life because they know best.

- I want to fit in at any cost.

- If other people say this food is good for me, then it must be true.

- I learn about my relationship to my body through observing how others relate to their bodies.

- If my mother/father love their body then I do too, but if they are always dissatisfied, then I think there is something wrong with my body also.

- I observe the people around me and learn that I am never good enough and my body is therefore never good enough.

- I follow the guidance of society to govern how much I weigh and what I eat. I allow the experts of the day and the cultural norm to govern my ideal weight and shape.

- I give up instinctive eating and body signals and eat as I am told I should be eating by the latest fads or according to research.

- Since I can't fit in I will rebel and eat badly in order to punish others.

STAGE 2: CONTROL

In the second stage of eating, you move on from simply following the lead of others to creating your own approach to eating, being, and moving, often based on controlling your body, your life, and your behavior around food. This stage is where you decide what is best for you. What you end up deciding will depend on what you have learned and kept from the copycat stage. It depends on what others have told you is best for you, and how you now use this information. For some of you, it will mean living a very controlled existence in relation to food and exercise, while for others it will mean giving up on yourself, seeing yourself as a failure, and punishing yourself as a result.

The control stage and way of being very much depends on a "right" and "wrong" approach, black or white. It depends on doing very particular things in order to get certain results, and the perceived success of your life becomes based on goals and outcomes. Goals and outcomes rule at this stage of your perception, because you are always striving to be a certain way, look a certain way, and even feel a certain way. You believe at this stage that the physical body is who you really are, and if you are not perfect on the outside, then you have failed and deserve little if any love. The control stage is also characterized by using external approaches to gain what you want, like the latest diet, pills, and exercise techniques. You believe these are all under your influence and control, and if you fail at looking good on the outside, then you have simply lost control and need to gain it back at any cost.

I have found from my many years of counseling clients that, funnily enough, this stage develops because in fact food and eating is perhaps the ONLY thing that people actually do have control over in life. You really do not have control over anything else at all. You cannot control what life brings, other people or even yourself, but you can control what you eat. It is the only area in life where you are in charge and can feel in complete control. Children do not get to control very much in their lives when they are very young, but they can refuse to eat something. You get to choose what you put into your mouth and into your body. Hence, how often, and what, you eat can reflect how in or out of control you are really feeling about the other aspects of your life. The one thing you can actually control (food intake) often reveals to you how you are genuinely relating to life itself.

Some examples of the type of thinking in this stage:

- My relative success or failure depends on having control over my body and my life.

- So long as I look good then I am a success in life.

- I have lost control if I gain weight.

- I have no control and no willpower if I am overweight.

- There is good and bad food and I need to avoid bad food and eat only good food.

- I must exercise in order to lose weight.

- I listen to the experts about what's good for me to eat or how to exercise.

- I follow the popular diet of the day rather than following my own instinctual intuitive eating approach.

- I do not trust my body. It wants to make me fat, so I need to control it.

- Since I do not have control over any other part of my life, I will control my food intake instead. That makes me feel in control of my life.

- I eat when, how and what I think I need to eat for fear of getting fat or sick.

STAGE 3: WHO AM I?

In this stage you begin to search for meaning. You begin to search for who you are in this world made up of success and failure. You look past the initial outside image of yourself and others and begin to look for who you really are. You begin to challenge old perceptions, moving beyond the universal "right" and "wrong" concept to find your own version of what is right and wrong for you as a unique individual. This stage is characterized by the ceasing of internal conflict. You stop fighting yourself and the world at this stage and instead seek to find who the real you is, in among all the conditioned parts of yourself developed during the copycat stage. You come to realize that no external thing ever had power over you and you take responsibility for being the creator of your own life. Hence, the search for your inner truth becomes the search for your true inner self. In regards to food and your body, you begin to ask questions such as, *"What do I really want to eat?" "What movements make me feel good?" "What does living in my body feel like?"*

The search in this stage is to find a place of inner peace rather than outer perfection. Ironically, the more inner peace one attains, the more "perfect" the outer self is given permission to be.

Some examples of the type of thinking in this stage:

- I am more than my body.

- I am safe to eat whatever I desire at any given moment.

- Listening to my needs and desires is important to do regularly.

- I love and appreciate myself and treat my body like a temple.

- How I think creates how I look and feel.

- I choose a movement form that nurtures me and is joyful to participate in.

- I take responsibility for my thoughts, beliefs, emotions, and actions. I can see why I sometimes make harmful choices and can choose to change this.

- I am perfect, whole and complete just as I am.

- I allow my body to choose its version of the perfect me rather than trying to force it, or to create it superficially.

- I am my best natural weight at all times.

STAGE 4: FINALLY FREE

The fourth and final stage of development is where you become finally free. In this stage you live completely and utterly as an independent being, understanding that you are here for yourself first and foremost. You love and nurture yourself unconditionally and perceive yourself, your body, and your life as free and unlimited. Your internal self is so full at this stage that there is no other choice but to share it with others, helping and serving from a place of love and acceptance rather than to gain the love and approval of others. At this stage you can finally be yourself. You understand that no external thing ever had any power over you. You listen to your body cues, follow your passions, and very little limits you. At this stage you realize you are part of something bigger than yourself. You see yourself as more than a physical body. You worship yourself as a piece of divinity on Earth and understand that spirit is what you are, first and foremost, for it enlivens all that you are. At this stage you follow nature and the rhythms of life. You ebb and flow in natural harmony and synchronicity and you have inner peace as the core part of your being. You are "finally free."

Some examples of the type of thinking in this stage:

- I am perfect just as I am.

- All food is perfect. All food is good. I choose what to eat with joy and inner knowing.

- I move for the sake of joy and balance.

- I am a reflection of life and divine perfection.

- I live in the freedom of knowing my body can be transformed without force and purely from my own intent.

- I am a powerful creator of my life and can create all that I choose.

- I show others the way to be free through being the change in myself.

- Food is pure joy.

- I follow my intuition in all ways.

- I am divinely perfect. Nothing else is true.

These stages have nothing to do with age. Your level of thinking will reflect how you relate to yourself, your body image, and your self-esteem. As you progress through the rest of this book, you will be led essentially from stage one into a stage four way of being and thinking. It is a natural progression, so all you need to do is allow it to happen and it will. It is also very normal to cycle through these. One minute it may feel as though you are genuinely at stage four and then all of a sudden you wake up and find yourself back in stage one. This too is normal. Cycling through these stages allows a deeper and deeper release of old ways of thinking each and every time, until finally you are at the place of feeling these changes within yourself and living them fully in your life. At this level of mastery nothing can ever take them away again.

As we undertake this process together, arm in arm, through the highs and natural lows, I encourage you to carry the following acronym with you: ANGEL.

A – Acknowledge your feelings

N – No judgment

G – Guilt free

E – Emphasize the positive

L – Let go

ACKNOWLEDGE YOUR FEELINGS

As you read this book, many feelings will emerge from within. It is important to acknowledge these feelings as they arise, because they are the doorway to change. Rejecting any feeling will only give it permission to fester and cause more negativity down the track. Acknowledge yourself if you feel frustrated, sad, angry, or resentful, and celebrate when you feel exhilarated, joyful, and peaceful. You don't need to do anything with how you feel. Just notice it. Awareness is the key to both balance and change in each moment.

NO JUDGMENT

Through judgment you will not progress very far in this or any other process. Self-judgment will bring you down and sabotage you. If you catch yourself thinking things like, *"Other people can do this, but I can't,"* don't take this as truth. Judgments are rarely true or helpful, so instead focus on being kind to yourself as you go through this phenomenal change process. Judgments can only harm you if you believe them or are unaware of them. As you become aware that you are judging yourself, then these judgments lose their power over you.

GUILT FREE

As you read this book, layers of guilt may emerge from you. Guilt is how most of us were socialized. Guilt is showing you that you feel bad for not being humanly perfect. The thing is, if you came to Earth to be humanly perfect, you have come to the wrong planet! It is impossible to be humanly perfect. Instead think of yourself as spiritually perfect, and remind yourself throughout this book that, so long as you do the best you can at any given moment, this is enough.

EMPHASIZE THE POSITIVE

As you progress through this book, always focus on your positive progress and successes. Doing this will provide a fertile environment for change to take place. See any setbacks or limitations as opportunities to break through your barriers and know that, no matter what, you always end up at the positive loving place within yourself. It always draws you back.

LET GO

When you feel challenged or feel fear rising in you, it is important that you do not attempt to resolve it. This may sound like a contradiction; however, your mind can never access the divine solutions that often await you. Letting your problems go instead allows something bigger and greater than your thinking to come to your aid. Let go when you get stuck and a solution will come to you. Surrender what feels too hard or impossible to solve, and it will be released on your behalf. In return the "how" will show up and often be miraculous in nature.

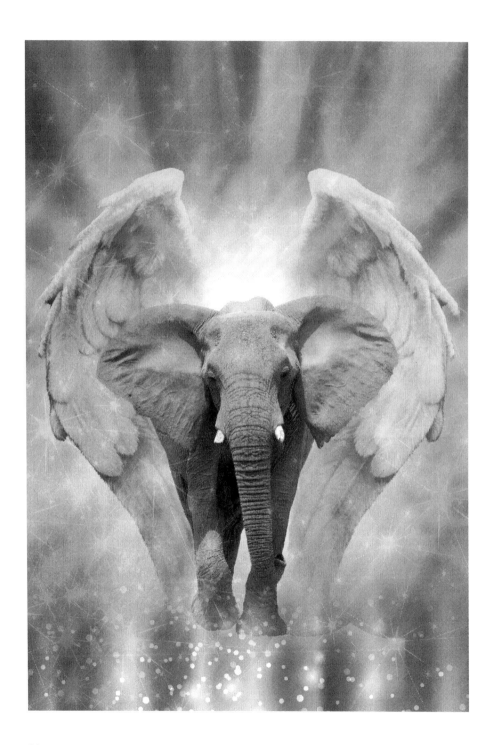

CHAPTER 2

CHANGE THE CONSCIOUSNESS
OF YOUR BODY

It is with great anticipation that I meet with you on this day to share the secrets of changing the consciousness of your body. I will be by your side for this adventure of inner growth and expansion. I will assist you to transform what you believe to be a solid body that operates within the rules that you have assigned to it. You will learn that you are free to alter these rules. Better still, you are free to make up your own rules.

What determines the consciousness of your body? Your body is a reflection of your mind consciousness. In other words, your body (and life) is merely a reflection of what you are thinking. In the book *The Key to Self-Liberation: 1000 Diseases and Their Psychological Origins*, Christiane Beerlandt describes, with uncanny accuracy and reflective depth, the true messages our bodies reveal about the way we currently think about ourselves and our lives. Detailing these 1000 diseases, she claims that inner healing "happens on the emotional and psychological levels, in the realms of emotions and convictions, or expectations, and of the image one has of oneself." These are the things that contribute to the consciousness of your body. Gregg Braden in *The Divine Matrix* points to research which now proves that how we feel influences the way the cells in our body function.

Hence, the consciousness of your body is a reflection of the consciousness of your mind and, more specifically, of your thoughts and feelings. Your body is a product of your mind. It is a common saying *"You are what you eat,"* but perhaps it ought to be *"You are what you think and feel."* Your body is a mirror back to you of your thoughts and perceptions. If you think something will make you gain weight, it will. If you believe you are not good enough, your body will communicate this back to you in some way. Therefore your body is always revealing to you what you are really thinking and feeling. In order to transform the consciousness of your body, you need to change your thoughts to a positive, new way of thinking that will affect your body positively too.

An undisciplined mind will easily and clearly be reflected in what appears to be an undisciplined body. The mind is vast. It holds a great deal of information within it. The subconscious mind brings forth into your consciousness beliefs that are made and stored primarily during childhood, and possibly even from throughout your family history. Whatever within you is not resolved lives on until you understand what it is there to teach you, at which point it can be released. Whether you are aware of it or not, the actions you take and the decisions you make in your everyday life are based on these deep-seated values and beliefs. They act as filters to your life choices and current life experiences.

Many of the profound spiritual leaders of our time suggest that you are not your past and you need not be governed by it. Instead they speak of the Divine or God as something to be found within you rather than outside of you. They relate, in a myriad of ways, that you are this living presence and that your past cannot be stronger than this truth. Assuming this to be true, why then does your conditioning and limiting past continue to rule you at times? Why are you so often limited through the "rules" you have adopted based on your past? It is common parlance in spiritual practices to speak of being in "alignment" with the Divine Being. This means essentially that you understand that God is within you and is stronger than anything from your past or any of your limited thinking. Yet this alignment happens through your own consciousness, through your subconscious and unconscious minds. Negative beliefs and filters in your subconscious mind will invariably block the flow of this divine knowledge and understanding that is waiting to operate through you. Divine guidance comes through you as the precious vessel that you are. In other words, you need to be a clear vessel in order to be in clear alignment with this greater power.

Divine Being is Divine Mind. Your mind is part of the Divine's energy and so is your body. Your consciousness was pure when you emerged from this source. You knew and remembered who you really were. Babies know and remember who they really are when they first arrive, until their parents and the world at large begins to condition them. When you came into your physical existence, you began to recognize yourself not as a part of the whole universal intelligence, but rather as a separate being. In forgetting who you really are, you set off to learn what you already know but have forgotten. Namely, you set off to learn how to live in love, freedom, and joy.

The truth, as I see it, is there is nothing that you really need to learn. You already know everything. Earthly experiences are your way of giving to the Earth, of playing on the earth plane, and engaging with consciousness itself. In other words you have come here for the mere experience and to have fun. Divine Mind always moves forward and grows in its wisdom and knowledge through your being here on Earth. Ultimately, you are only made of love and you will always return to the emptiness of mind, to the spaciousness of being, and to the true recognition of who you really are. You are headed to this place now. Everyone is headed there whether they realize it or not and will get there either willingly or kicking and screaming.

Life is full of seeming challenges. There appear to be many lessons to learn and many hardships to overcome in life. As you strive for peace, harmony, love, joy, spiritual connection, and wholeness of self, fear often gets in the way. Life appears full of fearful events, worries, and problems. Problems appear to be the way of the world. Problems appear on every corner, and life seems to be about always overcoming some type of problem. You carry many memories and wounds of problems from your past. You carry some emotional wounds that seem to stay no matter what technique is utilized to release them. Your brain remembers everything. There is nothing that can be forgotten, even if you cannot recall it. All of your wounds are fear-based memories.

When love is presented to you in its many guises, it often hits this wall of fear in you, and is not allowed to pass through the subconscious mind into the conscious mind. You are always measuring everything you see and do in relation to your wounds and endeavoring to be safe at all costs. Your one prerogative in life is to be safe in every way, by any means, no matter what is required, and no matter what it takes.

Safety is paramount to you.

Hence, from the moment you emerge as a human being, from other human beings who have come before, you are taught things to keep you safe in the world. Safety does not refer to escaping from a tiger charging toward you, although certainly this was the case in times gone by. Safety today means having enough money. Safety means being physically, mentally, and emotionally protected. Safety means being physically strong so you can protect yourself or at least have more prowess. Safety means feeling important, for if you are important and seen as important by others, you are indeed safe in the world. Safety means fitting in. Safety is shelter. Safety ultimately is love, hence why you go to such extreme measures to make sure you gain the love and approval of others. *"If others love me, then I am safe,"* or so you believe. Therefore any, and I mean any, reaction of the body, which is not of peace, wholeness, and harmony is a reflection of a mind that believes it is not safe. Lack of safety can reveal itself to you as tension, stress, anxiety, shame, guilt, fear, blame, jealousy, envy, anger, and many other forms.

Yet, the truth is, you are perfectly safe.

You may find yourself thinking *"I am not safe! Have you seen what is occurring financially in the world's economy? I am not safe. Have you seen how people are murdered, robbed, lose their money, lose their loved ones, lose all the things that are important to them through fires, wars, and so many other ways? Where is my safety?"*

"Have you seen in the schools how children taunt and tease each other? Have you seen in business how, if you are not smart enough, creative enough, talented enough, you are not considered important, or lose your job, or are not employed in the first place? Where is it safe in this world?"

Such statements are only too familiar. One only need watch the nightly news to see that the world clearly does not appear to be safe, by any means. Hence, we are constantly striving to become a "somebody" of importance, as though this will somehow magically make us safe in the world.

It is important at this point to remind you, the reader, that these are not just words on a page. That the very being and the essence of who you are—a divine creation on a divine earth in a divine body—is portrayed through and delivered to every cell in your body as you read and even as you hold these words. In fact, if you at any point give up reading the rest of this book, or if for whatever reason your mind cannot grasp the concepts in my words, try placing this book under your pillow at night and sleep upon it. In this way the meaning of all that is said and intended will help enter your being and further create the changes that you require. It can help bring your body and mind back to who you really are and back to truth. It will bring you back to your real inner self and erase all in you that is not true, including any false beliefs, thoughts, and emotions regarding how your body operates around food. It may seem like a silly thing to do, sleeping on a book and expecting this to do anything at all; however the premise of this technique is based on your infusion of the information and energy contained in the book. I have personally tried this many times with books, which I have found too complicated or exhausting to continue reading, and have been amazed at the subtle shifts that have occurred in me. While it may not be something you can actively measure in terms of results, it is still an exercise you may find useful. I offer it as a possibility.

This process is not overly complicated. You do not need pages and pages of theories about food, body weight, calories, and exercise. That, from this point of view, is pointless. The simple truths expressed in this book will set you correctly in motion and you will see the results, I assure you.

Your body is made up of cells and these cells are always in divine, perfect order. In other words they never do anything by accident. They are intelligent. It is commonly said that you are Spirit having a physical experience, but the truth is you are Spirit, full stop. Your body, your mind, your soul are all of spiritual essence. Just because you have taken form as solid matter does not imply that you are outside or separate from the rules or structures of Spirit. Your body is still of a spiritual nature, hence it is not separate from Spirit. It is a pure reflection of the whole Spirit that you are.

Think of your physical body as something that it is a mirror of how Spirit is expressing itself.

Yes, you are completely made of divine love energy. But when this love energy mixes with fear, a different color emerges. Taking this color example one step further, even though what was originally pure white now looks black, the white is still within the black. The color white has not gone, it is now simply hidden. Your body is the same. Just because your spirit cannot be seen, does not mean it is not there. It is and your understanding that it exists eventually brings it back to the forefront. Using our color example, through understanding the white is still in the black, you bring the white forward until one day you simply do not pay any attention to the color black and it therefore ceases to be influential. Hence, things that appear as problems initially likewise disappear when you begin to remember and reinforce that all you are is Spirit, first and foremost.

In the book *How God Changes Your Brain: Breakthrough Findings from a Leading Neuroscientist*, Andrew Newberg M.D. and Mark Robert Waldman investigate the effect that spirituality has on the brain and nervous system. They report that spiritual practices strengthen the anterior cingulate of the brain, which governs social awareness, intuition, and empathy. In strengthening the anterior cingulate of the brain, the activity of the amygdala slows down, the amygdala governing the fight-or-flight response in the body. They also speak of spiritual belief as decreasing the activity of the parietal lobes in the brain, which creates a feeling of being unified with the Divine or universe. God really does appear to change the brain!

Life does not require a choice or a battle between good and bad. There is no battle going on between the Love Self and the Ego Self. Love is all that really is and the ego is merely a false projection of your fear and ultimately a result of your separated thinking. This thinking has led you to create a self-image separated from the knowledge that you are Spirit first and foremost, and this source energy that you are is all that you are. The ego, as I see it, is not even real, and every time we feed it, we feed a totally false sense of ourselves.

Divine will, on the other hand, is required, for it puts Divine Being into divine action. In other words, when you are given inner guidance on how to best progress in your life, your will motivates you through to action. Your will is very important, hence why it exists. Allowed to run rampant, however, without divine inner knowing and without that higher source to guide it, will allows fear to overcome it and adopts beliefs and thoughts based on bringing about safety at any cost.

Ask yourself, therefore, in any given moment, is your thinking coming from your inner wisdom and knowing, or is it coming from that place of fear within you. I like to ask myself, *"Is my thinking coming from above or below me?"*

"Above" representing purity and "below" representing pure logic or fear. This is the sort of question you need to ask yourself often in order to bring your thinking back to truth. Remember, higher thoughts, or true inner wisdom, will feel as if it is coming from your higher self and from love. Such thoughts will appear neutral, unattached, and have a pure vibration. On the other hand if thoughts are coming from below the level of truth, they will be influenced by fear, a lack of safety in your body, a lack of safety in your life, and a lack of safety in your perception of the world.

Your only task, therefore, at this point in time, is to begin the process whereby your body, the mirror that it is, begins to receive a different, more positive reflection from the mind. Your body needs to be cleansed of the accumulated effects of your "fear thoughts" up until now. It needs to be cleansed of the desperate need, a need it believes is paramount, to keep itself safe at any cost. When this occurs it will know and remember the truth: that it is always safe because your thinking creates the world and not the other way around. Think thoughts of love and love is what you create. Think thoughts of war and war is what you create.

Interestingly enough, as you begin to embrace this concept in your life and spread your understanding of it to all areas of your life, you will also change the way you react to food. If the world is completely safe and there is nothing at all to fear, then this also holds true for food. Suddenly you are free to realize that all food is safe and neutral, and it is simply your thoughts that influence its effect on you. Really knowing and believing this, the body will no longer need to take any molecule of food and turn it into the structure of fat.

Fat is a God-given thing. You may not see it this way right now, but it is insulation that was given to you to wrap and protect you from thoughts, feelings, and emotions related to being unsafe in the world. You need not do anything to correct your appetite or eating habits. Please understand that when you have walked through all of the steps provided in this book, all of these things will be regulated, and hence, formed for their own sake and in their own way. My only concern here is having you feel safe. This alone will transform all aspects of your energy system including your chakra system, meridian system, auric fields, and all other finer energetic aspects. In so doing, this will bring balance and harmony to your physical body.

You do not need to forcefully change what you eat. This will change of its own accord in its own time, naturally and without effort. You do not need to undertake complex systems of exercise or diet. You only need to transform the mirror. In transforming the mirror, you align your Divine Mind to flow through to your human mind again. Be patient as you work through the various levels that this book has to offer you. Even if it does not make sense at times or seems too hard, it isn't. It is exceptionally simple and once you get it, you keep it forever!

THE "LOVE CORRECTION" VISUALIZATION

Do the following guided visualization to assist in beginning your transformational process. To undertake this meditation, please lie down anywhere it feels comfortable. If you need to, you may cover yourself lightly and hold the book and read it to yourself as you undertake this process, or listen to the audio version.

Imagine that in your left hand you have a clear quartz crystal. In your right hand you have a purple amethyst crystal. You don't need to really hold them. Feeling them in your imagination is enough. Bring your two hands together as if in prayer, bringing these two crystals into perfect union. Hold your palms together, allowing the crystals to merge.

Now place your right palm on top of the back of your left hand, left palm facing your body, bring them both into the space between your two physical eyes, touching your third eye. Hold them there for three seconds, then move them down to your throat. The palm of your left hand is still facing your throat, right palm on the back of the left hand, counting to three. Then continue to move your hands in this position to the chest area either where the heart is or in the center of the body where the heart chakra is. Count to three and move your hands on top of your navel in the same way. Keep your hands here, as the energy moves to the solar plexus (above the navel) and down to the sacral region (below the navel) and then back to the navel area where your hands still are.

When you are ready, move your hands down farther still, placing them over your pubic bone. Count to three and gently place your hands and arms by your side once again. When you are ready, turn over lying on your front. You may move your head to face one direction or the other, or you may prop yourself up on your arms. You will not be in this position for too long.

In this position your arms and hands may be wherever it is comfortable, your head in any way that feels right for you. Breathe in to the base of the diaphragm so that it feels as though you are breathing in to your lower stomach and breathe out through your mouth. Do this two more times, breathing in and breathing out, breathing in ... and breathing out. Now all you have to do is lie here. Just imagine as you lie here that a beautiful white light is moving through your brain and spinal area, removing all that is required, all of the things that are imprinted there that cause you fear.

Understand that this fear comes from the experiences you yourself have had in this lifetime, in other lifetimes, and through experiences that have been passed down to you through your family. In your brain, spine, and nervous system there is fear and lack of safety that is shared with all of mankind. There is also fear from the group consciousness of those long ago in the past that have been hurt, tortured, and even murdered for expressing certain beliefs and thoughts. Any fear of speaking your truth, fear of judgment, shame, and guilt from your lower spine leading up to the base of the skull is being erased. Continue to imagine this white light removing it all. As this is happening chant to yourself "Only God is in my mind," over and over again.

This erasing is occurring to the mirror which is your mind and this erasing is occurring to the physical body.

Rest assured that it is working whether you can feel something or not. Let it take as long as it needs to and give gratitude for the power that you have to create your own healing and balancing. You do not need me or any other healer to do this for you. Believe in yourself! You are powerful beyond measure. If I can do it for you better than you can do it for yourself, then this is only because I believe more than you do right now. Decide in this moment to believe in yourself and your healing power as much as I believe in you!

Your body from this day forth will no longer feel unsafe in the same way that it once did. Old imprints from all directions of time and space, through all levels of existence and dimensions, have been erased.

When you are ready you may turn and lie on your back again. Allow yourself now to imagine and even physically feel blue light entering your abdomen, cleaning and purifying all of the organs, all of the power centers of the body, all of the muscles and tendons. Imagine this blue light cleansing all of you. All of you. All of you.

Allow this light to now become an emerald green color. Green light is all that you are and all that you see. It is the color of healing, love, and peace. Stay in this green light for a few seconds. A repatterning is occurring. It matters not if you believe. This will work on anybody. It matters not if you believe. Know this. You do not need to believe yet. I believe in you and that is all that is required, remember. This is occurring within you right HERE AND NOW. Your mind is powerful and you are making this happen. I understand that you may not trust that this has occurred. Perhaps you are concerned that you will impress upon the body new issues tomorrow that will undo what has been done. This cannot be. You are now crystal clear.

Take some time to relax as you come back to yourself. Become aware of your breathing. Move your arms and legs and wake yourself back up. How do you feel?

After completing this meditation, do something that is fun and freeing, light and love-filled, something in this instance that has nothing to do with eating, at least for ten minutes following this advice. It is also helpful to drink some water.

You are now free of fear. You are now safe. You are now YOU.

CHAPTER 3

ALIGN FREE WILL WITH DIVINE WILL

Many of you yearn to be free of your obsession with food, and free of the unhealthy obsessions with your body. Unhealthy obsessions with your body can fairly easily manifest in a society constantly focused on health and well-being.

Divine Mind knows that your body is perfect, healthy, well, and slender, right here and now. Each of you is designed from within to be at the perfect weight and health for your body. Each of you has, within the perfect body system, a barometer built in, a set point to where the body returns in terms of weight and health when you allow it to do so. When you try to force the body to go where your mind believes it has to be, there is often a backlash effect which disturbs the equilibrium of your body. If you force the body to lose weight, starve yourself, limit what you eat, eat only certain foods, and engage in such obsessive behaviors, at some point the body will once again rebalance you by bringing cravings for the very things you were avoiding in the first place.

Your body knows how to be naturally thin. Your body knows how to release excess energy. Divine will is the mind of the universe and includes all that exists in harmony together. From this place, information is harmonious and peaceful, united and serene, strong and powerful. From this place, you are seen as being only one thing—a divine being. From this place within yourself, you understand the true nature of food. You cannot see this, however, when your free will is not united with divine will, universal will, and nature. In order for this to occur, you need to surrender and trust your body and life. Trusting yourself and feeling at peace with all food is the result when these levels of being are united within you.

Free will is part of universal law, which gives you the right, freedom, and the ability to choose your own way through life. It provides you with the opportunity to choose how to think, be, feel, respond to, and perceive the world around you. It provides you with the ability to make whatever choices you believe are best, to choose the beliefs that serve you, and to choose your life path. You are free to live as you see best, hence all that comes to you in life comes from your own making. Your choices and actions are a reflection of what you think, believe, and feel.

You are therefore granted the ability to choose what to believe and how to think and feel about food, your life, and your body in terms of health, well-being, and weight. If you have a belief that a certain food will make you gain weight, or that a certain food is bad for you, then you create this to be so.

Free will gives you this power, but it also gives you the negative effects of your beliefs, thoughts, emotions, and ultimately your choices and actions. Free will, while being a magnificent gift, giving you the ability to live your life as you choose, also requires that you take full responsibility for whatever you attract into your life. You are the one producing the effects that come to you. All things relate back somehow, even when not initially obvious, to your mind, your thoughts, and to the way you engage with the world.

Thus far, your logical, biased thinking has led you to believe so-called experts and scientific studies as the foundation on which to base your decisions. You are convinced that others know more than your innate wisdom, than your intuitive thinking. Science has educated you to believe that you need to undertake a certain amount and type of exercise, eat certain foods, and avoid unhealthy foods in order to lose weight. This is the power of your free will, to choose what and who you believe.

You may have incorrectly assumed that overweight people are hopeless, lack will power, and that there is something wrong with them, or with you. It is certainly not seen as desirable to be overweight, and those that are face humiliation and judgment from others. You are deemed a failure, either by yourself or by others, when you have allowed yourself to become overweight. *"If I had just listened to the 'experts' this wouldn't have happened,"* is often the deep-seated belief.

Some of you may have given up altogether on trying to lose weight, on trying to be healthy, or even trying to gain weight. You have tried again and again, and every time you judge yourself as having failed, you believe that you are weak instead of strong. You are a prisoner of your own beliefs, limited by your own mind, and limited by your inability to use your free will to your advantage. You are possibly following the examples of your parents, friends, or society at large. You may blame yourself for not being strong enough, well enough, slim enough, or beautiful enough. You have blamed yourself for so much.

You try to find your way back through this one magical word to which you are a slave—CONTROL! You believe that if you lose control, then you are a failure. *"I had complete control over my life and then I lost it." "I was in control of what I ate, but now I have lost control and I need to get it back."* This is the sort of self-talk you engage in, perhaps, as though to suggest that your body took over and broke down and took control away from you. You believe your body does not support you, but the truth is you do not support the beautiful, vibrant, living organism, which is your body. It is your support that is required, and not your body's support of you. Your body just follows your orders. Control is nothing but an illusion. The more in control you appear to be, the more fearful you are of losing control, thinking that through its loss your entire life will fall apart. Hence, you try to control yourself, others, and even the environment.

Control is simply a safety measure. You believe it is necessary in order to keep what you have and to gain all that you desire. You are told time and again, in regards to health, if you do not maintain control of your health through taking vitamins and minerals and forcing your body to exercise in the latest ways, that you are not good enough. You may think you are living the best life your free will allows, but this is in fact control in disguise. This is imprisoned will, for it acts from the rules and regulations and the laws of a mind that has forgotten itself—a mind which is fearful and in panic. What is the good of living life if you fear it all the time? What is the good of eating food if you fear the consequences of it all the time? What is the point of eating something just because someone else tells you it is good for you? You have convinced yourself of so many untruths. So many lies you have believed and continue to believe. The only person with truth and wisdom, however, is YOU.

You are not your body. You are not your beauty. You are not your weight. You are not the food you eat.

You are only the thoughts you think and the feelings you feel.

Do you know that thoughts are directly related to the acupuncture meridians in your body, hence negative thoughts about food, body, health, weight, and all other things create negative blockages in these meridian pathways? In my experience, it is blockages in the meridians that can directly cause physical illness and inability to heal from injuries. This is why Chinese medicine is regarded as one of the most ancient and successful healing practices. If thoughts really do block your meridian channels and cause disturbances in your physical body, potentially hindering weight loss, then imagine if you have an estimated sixty thousand thoughts in a day, how many blockages you must have?

One very powerful way to overcome such blockages and allow yourself to return to your inherent wisdom and the highest use of your free will, is to reconnect your free will with your divine will. In doing this, you recognize there is a higher power and you allow it to operate through you, as you. In *The Divine Matrix*, Gregg Braden describes divine will: "The Divine Matrix [is the container that] holds the universe, the bridge between all things, and the mirror that shows us what we have created." Since your divine will is a template for perfect thought and action, aligning with it brings you back to the highest good in yourself. Held in alignment long enough, the grid which is your physical system and the information that feeds and informs this grid also alters permanently. Aligning with divine will allows the higher order of who you are to flow through you in each and every moment, allowing universal truths to influence your life. These universal truths can overlay and overcome your limiting beliefs. When you are aligned in this way, you always inherently know what is best for you to eat at any given moment in time. You do not have to rely on guessing, bad choices, or the voices of so many others in your head. You have the ability to choose and transform, at will, yourself and all that you eat. You remember your inherent spiritual power. You remember yourself and who you really are.

Coming back to the book mentioned earlier, *How God Changes Your Brain: Breakthrough Findings From a Leading Neuroscientist* by Andrew Newberg M.D. and Mark Robert Waldman, through the use of brain scan technology they were able to see that blood flow and electrochemical activity in many areas of the brain changed according to various feelings and thoughts. Thoughts and feelings really do alter the brain activity! Even more amazing was the effect of thinking about God or spiritual practices, such as meditation, on the brain. Positive outcomes included enhanced cognition, communication, and creativity. Spiritual practices were even found to "change our neurological perception of reality itself." Perhaps one day in the not so far future, research will focus on how this shift in perception of reality alters the body itself and its ability to lose weight.

All food begins as neutral energy. Food is inherently neither positive nor negative. Positive or negative information is given to food through the consciousness of the human mind. If the human mind decides that food is negative, then this is what it becomes. If a person believes that meat is wonderful and positive, then this is what it becomes, whereas if they believe it is harmful, then this is what it becomes for them. All food begins as neutral and your body is always whole and healthy and well. You mind is always connected to your heart, to your gut, to source, to divine knowledge, to the Earth, to nature, to the wisdom of the universe and the entire planetary realm. I am reminded of infamous Chinese masters recorded in history as being able to ingest cyanide poisoning and not be affected. Certainly they did not die. Why? Perhaps they knew how to relate to it as a neutral substance.

'WHO I REALLY AM' EXERCISE

State out loud every chance you get, and particularly when you feel out of alignment, the following statement to instantly return to your divine will operating through you, and as you:

"I know who I am. I am the Divine in all my being, hence the truth is that my will is the divine will. They are one and the same. I am not separate from my will. As I trust and have faith in myself, I know that my free will becomes well-guided. I surrender this thing called control that comes from fear in my mind, as well as old fears trapped in my body. I know I am safe now. I understand that I am working through this process, and with each passing day, my alignment is more whole and complete. I am enriching my relationship with food, my body, and my perception of myself, and I enrich my entire life and so it is. I give thanks on this day and I know this to be so NOW."

CHANGE YOUR BRAIN WITH GOD VISUALIZATION

As you close your eyes, feel yourself glowing from the inside out. Imagine you are heating up as the energy emerges from the center of your body out through your entire being. At this moment in time, imagine you are the sun. You are the sun! As the sun, begin to observe the planets moving around you. Imagine that you are the one that gives them life. You are the giver of life. Imagine if the sun believed it wasn't good enough? Imagine if the sun believed it didn't belong. Imagine if the sun believed it was too big, too fat, too greedy, too weak, or had no purpose or power. Imagine if the sun decided there was no point in shining anymore and turned itself off. What would happen to all those that rely upon the sun? You are the sun at this very moment in your life. You are just like the sun on planet Earth to many others. You are the sun to the plants and the animals and to other human beings. When you think in negative ways it is like deciding to turn yourself off and in that moment you destroy yourself. So shine right now. Shine and decide that you will stay the sun no matter what. Decide that you will love yourself no matter what. Give yourself a hug here and now as you sit. You are the sun.

Take a deep breath and now imagine you are the moon. Feel yourself glowing, luminous, filling up the night sky. You are the moon. What would happen if the moon suddenly decided there was no point hanging around in the sky anymore? What would happen if the moon fell out of the sky? You are the moon. The energy of the moon affects all of life on Earth. You are the moon to so many people in your life. Nature and the animals require you. Smile to all of your body, including your internal organs. You are the moon.

Now imagine you are Earth. You are home to so many. You are nature itself. You are the Earth. Feel this in your core. What would happen if as Mother Earth you suddenly decided you had enough of dealing with all the negativity poured upon you? What would happen if you grew tired of humans and couldn't bear the heat of the sun that suddenly grew hotter? What would happen if you suddenly stopped loving and gave up? What would happen? All the people, animals and plant life rely on you. They too would be gone, based on your choice. But, as the Earth, you gladly take the pain of those that inhabit you and gladly heal yourself and them. You are Earth at this moment. Allow yourself as Earth to send love, healing and blessings to all the people in your life whose Earth you are. Choose in this moment to live. In choosing to live, choose to allow your free will to align wholly and completely with your divine will. It is done. Take a deep breath and return afresh and new, as a new you.

CHAPTER 4

RELEASE PAIN FROM THE PAST AND ANXIETY FROM THE FUTURE

Do not be concerned with your progress so far. I encourage you to keep going no matter how much you have understood or feel you have changed. There is no need to stop after each chapter and analyze, judge, or fear your old self. This is unnecessary and will only hinder your journey. It will take longer this way. Just imagine, for the sake of imagining, that you are playing a game. Imagine you are five years old being taken on this journey, and you blindly, willingly, and even naively follow. Be five. Trust. Have faith. Believe.

I have touched upon the fact that your beliefs form a filter through your sub-conscious mind that filters information through to your conscious mind and out into the world and to your body. Your body and the world are but mirrors, which reflect all that you believe, think, and feel. This is perhaps an overwhelming realization, given that it probably feels to you that, on the whole, you are not really free to choose what you think. In the course of a day you rarely freely choose your thoughts, but rather it feels that they choose you. The past is largely what contributes to these thoughts and to the beliefs you hold about yourself, your body, your life, your relationships, your successes, your friends—EVERYTHING.

Beliefs are big influences. It is your beliefs that contribute to anxiety, fears about the future, what it holds, what it brings and how you will fare in the world. You are often anxious about whether you will be safe, whether you will be all that you came to be, whether you will fulfill your purpose, and whether you will be a beneficial presence on the planet. Perhaps you have anxiety about what lies ahead and death is your greatest anxiety of all. Let me not forget the anxiety about gaining weight, which presents to you each and every day! These are all forms of pain that you try to avoid in your life.

Pain, wounds, and limiting beliefs all come from your mind, which records the past and the experiences you have perceived. I want to challenge you that the only real pain is that you are here in the first place. Your only real pain is that you are on Earth. In having come here, you experienced a separation from your true identity and your true power. You are really the Divine Presence in human form. It is not arrogant to think this, but indeed humbling. The only sinful thought you have ever had was to think that you are not a piece of the Divine Presence and that you will never be good enough no matter how hard you try. This thought is the real pain, and it is this thought that, like a magnet, attracts into your life the experiences of fear, blame, guilt, shame, and all lower vibrational forms of emotions, beliefs, and negative thoughts.

When your beliefs, thoughts, and emotions all align, then you manifest that which you feel, think, and believe. They align to create what you want as though it is here already, right HERE AND NOW. This is the basis of manifestation. Nothing more needs to be done. This is also why many of you fail to manifest. For, without this combination of aligned beliefs, thoughts, and emotions, you cannot fully, easily, and effortlessly create what you desire.

In order to be whole and balanced in relation to your body, food, weight, and all things related to them, it is imperative that you believe that the world is safe, and you are safe in it. I have already spoken about this in Chapter 2, but now we are touching upon a crucial belief related to this:

You and the Divine are one and the same and have never been separate from each other. No separation ever occurred. When you were born on Earth, you did not separate from source energy.

Gregg Braden, in *The Divine Matrix*, states that within each of us "there's an unspoken sense that we're somehow separated from whomever or whatever is responsible for our existence." Yet we are not. He goes on to share evidence that comes from translating our DNA into ancient Hebrew and Arabic alphabets, which literally reads "God/Eternal within the body." This may be challenging for some of you to believe, but then it is probably unlikely that you would have picked this book up in the first place if you do not have a mind that is open to everything. The Divine Presence is not somewhere else waiting to be beckoned, pleased, bargained with, or waiting for you to earn its love, approval, or forgiveness. This divine source in all of its magnificence is within you. You are "it" and so are all others. Every time you insult yourself, every time you engage in lower vibrational thinking, you are deeply insulting that which you hold in such high regard: the universe, source energy, God.

You are a part of the whole and the whole is part of you. Hence you are a piece of the universe and the universe is a piece of you. You are one and the same. This is what we shall correct on this day. Correcting your belief in a separation that never existed will instantly erase all pain and wounds and all beliefs that limit you, in all directions of time.

Perhaps this is too simple. You may be wondering how this relates to food, but this book is about more than just food. Food represents life and living. Food represents your health, well-being, and peace of mind. All other areas of your life are reflected in your relationship to food. When you do anything in relation to eating, food, or body weight, you are essentially healing the whole person and bringing yourself back to the correct and true perception of who you really are.

Let me ask you this before we continue. If God were indeed one special being somewhere else, does God eat? Perhaps. Does God get fat? Does God hurt Itself? Punish Itself? Persecute, limit, and judge Itself? I believe not. God is all-knowing, perfect, complete harmony, peace, and perfection in all ways. Given that the being we speak of as God is essentially who you are, then you are these things also.

Remind yourself of this. Remind yourself of this often and you will be well pleased with yourself. You will find great shifts occur easily and readily. Such great shifts cannot be produced by any other human method or technique.

Only remembering WHO YOU REALLY ARE can bring about the permanent shift you seek.

It is the way of the psyche to always expand. It is the way of the world for human consciousness to grow to new frontiers. Everyone laughed when it was suggested the world was round, and people were once burned for having psychic abilities. Yet these new abilities and discoveries have always been available. Such expansion has only ever come from higher sources of being.

THE ROLE OF EMOTIONS

Let me now speak about emotions and the important role they play in triggering the body's reaction to food, craving for food, and use of food as self-punishment, and in many other ways that do not serve you. Candace B. Pert, PhD in her book *Molecules of Emotion* has changed the way we view emotions and their relationships with the body. She revealed mind-blowing evidence to support the fact that the mind affects emotions and emotions affect the mind. They are connected.

Your chakra system was gifted to you. It is just as important and inherent in you as your heart. You believe that you are alive because your heart beats, but there have been documented cases in the world where people's hearts have stopped beating, yet they continue to live. Your chakra system is just as important if not more so, in my view, than your heart. It informs your heart. It informs your other organs. It informs your body. Your chakra system informs the physical, hence it is critically important that it be kept in balance.

Balance looks like this: clean open chakras, which are emotionally at 100 percent in their capacity to deal with stress.

When the chakras are in balance something miraculous happens. When they are functioning correctly, you are free to feel all that you feel, positive and negative. A healthy-functioning chakra system that feels all things, and is permitted by the mind to do so, will process all emotions while permitting no scarring, no wounds, no trauma, no hurt to any of the chakras or to the body itself. Each chakra knows what area it governs and what feelings it is in charge of releasing. I will not go into each chakra in depth, as many books have been written on these topics. Here is a very brief summary of each:

- The crown chakra is located on the crown of the head and is to do with forgiveness and higher-world connection.

- The third eye chakra, located in the middle of the two eyes, manages higher vision and inner knowing.

- The throat chakra, located in the throat region, is related with creative self-expression and feeling that one is being heard.

- The heart chakra, located in the heart area of the body, deals with grief, loss, love, healing, and peace.

- The solar plexus chakra, located above the navel, deals with willpower, happiness, and joy.

- The sacral chakra, below the navel, is connected with relationships, decision making, sex, money, and food!

- The base chakra, located at the base of the spine, deals with safety and security and the bringing of one's creative energy to reality through taking action.

When things appear to go wrong or challenges appear and life unfolds in ways that you were not expecting, all sorts of emotions well up in you. Depending on what area of the body they relate to and which of the chakras they are connected to, there will be differing side effects. Emotions are not your enemy, although you sometimes run from them. Emotions are a gift. I repeat—they are a gift. They are your way to clear yourself of difficult life events. Feel what you feel—all of it. Feel every little bit of it and allow your chakras to process this information just as they were designed to do. When you allow all emotions to be processed by healthy chakras, there are no side effects.

It is the denial or inability to fully express all of your emotions that blocks chakras in the first place.

One of the most common side effects of blocking the chakras in this way is a cloudy and unclear intuition. Intuition is available to all of us through three major areas in the body, namely the gut, the heart, and the head. Intuition was not given to a few select people like me so that I could heal others. Intuition belongs to every single person, whether they choose to use it or not. It is rarely wrong and always available. I do what I do with unerring accuracy in seeing illness in the body because I listen to my intuition and I have trained it accordingly.

In an energetically, physically, emotionally, mentally, spiritually healthy being that recognizes their inherent spiritual perfection, the intuition of the heart, gut, and head work in perfect unison. This is why the triangle symbol is such a powerful symbol. This is why some approaches that are successful in health often call for the triad of health, meaning three different approaches—one for each of the head, heart, and gut. Likewise, practices that address these three areas are always more successful than practices that only deal with one of them. What you eat is relevant from the gut perspective. What you feel about what you eat is relevant from the heart perspective, and what you believe or think about the qualities of what you eat is relevant for the head or mind.

Today's journey will be to weave all three together—the mind, heart, and gut. You will clear all three channels for perfect grace and divinity and perfect communication and balance. Before you do this, allow me speak to you about the Cycle of Purpose.

THE CYCLE OF PURPOSE

Purpose is something you will search for at some point in your life. Purpose is connected to seeking a deeper meaning in life and finding true happiness on Earth. There are three phases to purpose.

The first phase of purpose is simply to BE.

You are here just to be. To exist. This is all you are required to do and be. Your existence on Earth makes a profound difference to all things. If a leaf is missing from a tree, you may not notice it, but the tree knows, for each leaf is relevant and unique. In the same way, your existence here creates important vibrational energy. Even though you may not have achieved anything significant, or you may not think you are anything special, each of us is uniquely special and all of us have fulfilled our purpose through just being here. This is the first aspect of your purpose.

The second phase of your purpose is to GIVE.

This is why you are driven so strongly to support, help, give, and be of service. This does not, however, mean serving others at your own expense. It does not refer to helping or saving others blindly as this will ultimately cost you. This sort of service is false service. The motivation for such service usually comes from seeking love and approval from others.

The service I speak of is of you functioning as a full being of love. If you have spent sufficient time appreciating and accepting the first phase of purpose, knowing that just being here on Earth is fulfilling your purpose, then you will already feel like a full cup of life, ready to spill over and naturally help others. If you truly understand that to BE here really is enough, then you will understand that no matter what has been done to you by another, or what you have done to another human being, none of these things have affected you. You are still perfect. All that is required is that you forgive yourself.

It follows that, in helping others, you serve because you are so full. You are a cup spilling over and what would you do with all this extra energy and love but contagiously share it with the world? Importantly, you share it through your unique talents, rather than in ways that others may want or expect of you. Unifying your heart intuition, gut intuition, and mind intuition contributes to the creation of amazing ways to help others, while also simultaneously helping yourself.

The third aspect of your purpose is pure FUN and PLAY.

You must serve first (in phase two) because the heart sings when it serves. First, you must serve because it is a profound awakening that lifts you out of the place of just being here. You want to assist the Earth you live on and its people. It is a desire inherent in you. Second, when you feel content from having given so much of yourself, then you need to play and replenish yourself. This too is part of your purpose—to play and experience life. Many of you find it very difficult to play, have fun, and be joyously frivolous without first having given of yourself. The serving and the being that come before this stage will make you feel so rich and help you remember who you really are, so when you play, you will not play falsely or egotistically, nor will you pretend to play. From this place, you will not play to be better than others or to prove anything. You will just play. Play can be whatever it is for you, a joyful and special time just for you. It is about serving your self. Self-giving. Self-nurturing. Self-growth.

Then one returns again to the first phase of the cycle—that of simply being here on Earth. This cycle continues on for eternity. This cycle is exceptionally important. It operates minute to minute. It operates in an hour, in a day, in a week, in a month, in a year, in a lifetime. You will see this cycle . . . always. If you pay attention to it and follow its lead you will find your life takes place with great ease.

If you find your head in a cookie jar (not because you know you can eat what you like and you are changing the consciousness of your body) because you are miserable, unhappy, feel as though you are wasting your life away, or because all of your life feels wrong, then come back to this cycle of purpose.

Start always at the first aspect of purpose in the place of being, accepting that you are enough just by being here. Just be. In this being place, know that you are enough. Nothing more is required of you. You are wonderful. Even if you spent all of your life in this phase, you are wonderful. You are so important. Your presence is so valued. Thank you for coming. Thank you for your great service of being here. Start in this place. Remember you will go through this cycle in small ways throughout a day and in much broader ways throughout a lifetime. Pay attention to it. It will set you free from many aspects in your life and is very relevant to food and your use of food to escape your destiny and purpose.

Ask yourself what phase in the Cycle of Purpose are you in today?

Let me now get to the real work of cleaning things up within you, of creating this transformation of your being, of releasing you from the pain of your past and the anxiety of your future, with the exercise below.

THE RELEASE CYCLE

If you allow it to be so and it feels right for you, close your eyes and imagine yourself standing in a beautiful field of rainbow-colored flowers. There are hundreds of different varieties and colors of flowers everywhere. You cannot see beyond them in the field. They are in such abundance. The sky above you is blue with beautiful trails of white clouds as though they have been gently painted with an angelic paintbrush.

The grass below your bare feet is cool and fresh, soft and velvety, and the flowers surrounding your ankles tickle you. Breathe the fresh air . . . . Breathe the fresh air . . . . (long pause)

Why the long pause you may ask? You are just being in this place. You are just as important as one of these flowers. Yes, you heard me right. You are just as important as they are.

From within the flowers that surround you, there are flowers disguised as flowers, but they are not flowers at all. They are aspects of your wounded self, of your pain, of separation from Divine Mind. Allow them now to reveal themselves. Notice what you see, feel, hear, and know. If you cannot visualize or see them revealing themselves, do not fear. They are presenting themselves nonetheless. TRUST.

Allow now the gentle breeze to blow the dark ones away. Well, perhaps the breeze is not quite so gentle at all. Perhaps it is a gust of wind that blows them far away to the point of erasing them from this universe, disintegrating them from time and space.

Allow fresh beautiful flowers to now grow in their place. Strong, new flowers. Good flowers. Now, as you stroll along the flowers, you come to a vegetable patch and you are suddenly overtaken with a desire to dig up some of these vegetables. Do so now. Pick as many vegetables as you desire, for you will be giving these away to the ones that you love and to the people that you believe require special love and care.

Simply ask that these vegetables give what others require from them. You are now in the phase of serving. You are serving just for the sake of it, because it feels good, because it feels right. These vegetables are your creative energy. Do not fear. Giving them away does not mean you give away your creativity. Giving them away means you have brought your creativity to each part of you now, and you are so full of wonder, what is there to do but share it with others? You are sharing your fully activated, free flowing, enthusiastic, inspirational creativity.

Now, dear one, notice that you have grown wings. Now you are a fairy just for the fun. Fly! You are living the third aspect of your purpose. Fly, and as you fly, travel beyond the divide, from your world to other worlds and see that it is no different. In fact, perhaps what you find is the farther you fly, the greater and cleaner the energy becomes. Fly, dear one, fly! Fly directly into the light and become one with it. Do not fear that in this light form you lose yourself. You will always know yourself.

Is this fun? Are you enjoying yourself. This is your fun time. Your play time. As you emerge blessed and cleansed and joyful, know there is nothing to fear. You will remember that you are special and worthy.

You will remember on a cellular level who you are. You will remember who you really are! **You will remember who you are from this moment forth, forever!**

Allow yourself to be surrounded by a swirl of light—a swirling action that runs counter-clockwise, cleansing all the grid systems that surround you, cleaning away old information, old pain, and anxiety. All of it. Any of it. All information that is irrelevant to the coherence of your true self, and to the coherence of your perfect alignment with the planet. All that is against or withdrawn from the perfect balance of your heart, gut, and mind being in perfect communication with each other is now erased. It is transformed into love and sent to others to help them do the same.

This will take a few more moments as it swirls around you in a counterclockwise fashion. You may feel tingling in your hands and feet as this is occurring.

Breathe deeply.

When you arise from this transformative practice, it is advised that you go and kiss yourself in the mirror. Yes, literally, go and find a mirror and kiss yourself. Look yourself deep in the eyes and say the following words:

"I remember who I am and I believe it. In fact, I know it to be true. And so it is."

"I remember who I am, and I fully believe it. I know it to be true. And so it is."

You only need do this meditation once. However if you enjoyed it, you may do it again. Go on, skip ahead. There is more fun to be had. More changes to be made. More to be gained. I skip along with you. I rejoice with you and for you. As you make this change, you give permission for others to do the same.

CHAPTER 5

THE TRUTH ABOUT FOOD

Food is sacred medicine. Food is medicine of the universe passed on to those of the Earth. Food is medicine of the Earth passed on to those of the Earth. It can be used for good and it can be used for harm. Its inherent power is in its use. Like all medicine it holds power, but the power in the medicine of food is more than it appears on the surface level.

The primary reason you eat is for health and vitality. You eat primarily to gain the correct vitamins, minerals, amino acids, and so forth that ensure your body grows well, regenerates, recuperates, and thrives. You eat first and foremost to be strong and vibrant, full of energy and vitality. In the Western world there are many food choices that are thought of as unhealthy. Foods, for example, that contain trans fatty acids, sugar, even carbohydrates have been called unhealthy of late. What is good to eat today and will help you lose weight may no longer be the trend tomorrow. Foods such as coconut oil and olive oil were once believed to cause weight gain and needed to be avoided, and now the experts tell us that coconut oil and olive oil are important for weight loss. There is so much contradictory information and so many contradictory results of numerous studies carried out. Some people eat a high quantity of food all day and do not gain weight, while others barely eat a thing all day and still gain weight. Others again find it a fight between staying slim and staying healthy, as though these are mutually exclusive.

So what new light will I shed on this matter today? The truth in my experience is we all have the ability to turn anything in life into neutral energy and even into positive energy. Since everything in the world is energy in its basic form, it can be changed. However, you also have the ability to transform positive energy into negative energy, and although this is rarely desirable, you are doing this more often than you think. According to Master Lin, founder of Spring Forest Qi Gong, an ancient Chinese healing art, "Everything is energy in different forms and there is not really good energy or bad energy until we think of it as good or bad." I love the way Master Lin describes all energy as "good, better, best" instead of good or bad. Imagine thinking of all food in this way!

I want to provide you with more than just some simple techniques to suppress your appetite, to change how you eat, or to make you finally stick to a healthy eating plan. I understand that you have probably tried every single diet that was ever thought up, only to go back to overeating and eating all the wrong things.

What if finally there was a way to eat anything you want and as much as you want and to know that you can transform what you are eating to be healthy, vibrant, and life-giving? In effect, imagine having the power to neutralize all negative information and then transform it into the positive. Energy can never be made or destroyed. Energy can only be transformed. So by neutralizing food you erase all of the information that it contains, and then you can give it positive energy, essentially bringing it into complete alignment with divine energy.

Divine energy has no polarity of good or bad. Divine energy is pure power, only good, only love. It is based on the positive and on love, has no fear and no negativity within it. There is only ONE POWER and that power is only the good in everything. Everything else that appears not to be good is just an illusion of the mind, based on the fear I spoke of earlier. This thinking approach is a giant step above the thinking of duality and polarity. Yes, you live in a world where polarity exists, but the truth of who you are is not based on this version of reality. Polarity was created through the mind and through judgment. So by eradicating the judgment you have placed on all foods and bringing them all back into the light of neutral and positivity within them, you will gain great discernment. Discernment will allow you to eat what your body, mind, and soul truly require at any given moment, knowing that it does not matter if it happens to be a burger or a salad—they are all one and the same. One and the same. Remember to think in terms of "good, better, best." Nothing is bad for you.

How is this even possible, you may ask? It is possible because you are a change agent. You have the ability to transform all energy. You have always had this ability. It hasn't just been given to you now. It's your latent gift. How much of your brain is not utilized? You are born with the potential to use all of it. Children understand this much better than adults. In fact, how many parents complain that children eat too much junk food, or at least want to? The error is not that they eat in this way. The error is that they are constantly told that they will not grow as a result of eating this way and told they will get sick and are being unhealthy.

If this does end up happening, we say, "I told you so," not recognizing that we may be the ones that planted the seeds of this occurring in the first place. Despite being nagged, children generally still continue to eat junk food, but now they have a set of beliefs about how bad this is for them, which will potentially cause more ill health in the future. This bad feeling will eventually become guilt as they grow, and then self-judgment, until eventually they fulfill their parents' prophecy of being overweight and unhealthy. Not because of the food, let's be clear, but because of the beliefs that were attached to it.

In his groundbreaking book, *The Hidden Messages in Water*, Masaru Emoto points out that absolutely everything vibrates at its own frequency. Words and intentions whether spoken or written display vibrations. According to Dr. Emoto, "water faithfully mirrors all vibrations created in the world," hence "when water is shown a written word, it receives it as vibration, and expresses the message in a specific form."

He photographed ice crystals that were shown words, sent various intentions, or played various types of music. The results were outstanding, showing the most divine organized crystalline structures from positive words and intents, and disturbed crystals from intent and words that were negative. Whatever you say and think—anything and everything that you think—becomes your reality and becomes true for you. Think *"This chocolate cake is going to make me gain weight tomorrow,"* and guess what will happen? You did that, not the chocolate cake. You must understand that the information imprinted into food does not come from you alone. Who prepared that chocolate cake? What were they thinking about it? Who handled each of the ingredients, and what thinking did they put into them? Love? Fear? Anger? Greed? Were they thinking of overweight people eating this cake as it was being made? All of this and more is in this chocolate cake. If the majority of the population thinks that chocolate cake is fattening, then this information, too, is in the chocolate cake. Perhaps this feels as if you are fighting a battle you cannot win, but you are not fighting a battle. I am asking you to begin being a conscious filter. You are a filter anyway, but be conscious now and intentional, and discover the power within you.

You can change any food into neutral energy, into God energy, into love energy, light energy, divine energy—into perfection. Doing this renders it safe, vibrationally clean, vibrationally high, and of a pure quality, life-giving, and health-giving. Any shadow of a doubt and you will not have neutralized it, nor empowered it. If you do not believe me, all you have to do is try it and see for yourself. See how you feel after you follow the technique that I will teach you in a moment to neutralize all food. You will do this exercise every day. If you do this every day for a year, which may seem like a long time (but it only takes a minute or two each day) you will develop a completely different relationship to food.

You needn't go live with monks on a mountaintop and bless all your food. Those monks know how to do this, but if they can do it, so can you, only differently and even more efficiently. All knowledge is universal knowledge and it belongs to all who wish to learn the secrets of utilizing energy. If it matters to you, then you can do it. If you forget to do this with any food you eat, it does not matter. You will do this for a year because it will train your energy system, your body, and your mind, until eventually every cell of your body, mind, and being will do it naturally, without conscious thought. It does not mean you will not feel the effects for a whole year however. You need to be conscious about it for the year to ensure the effects, and after this time the effects will occur on their own. Then it will be an unconscious event and be done for you automatically. Remind yourself that food is only energy by remembering Einstein's famous formula of $E=mc2$ which demonstrates that matter and energy are really just the same thing. Energy can be turned into matter and matter into energy!

THE UNIFICATION PROCESS®

If you are right-handed, then in the right hand imagine holding the energy of neutral energy, God, the One Power, Love, or whatever other name you wish to give it. In this hand you are holding the energy and information of pure divine perfection. There are no problems here, nothing to be fixed. If you are left-handed, you will hold this intent in your left hand.

In your other hand, imagine holding the problem that you wish to erase, or the food you wish to neutralize and make positive. In neutralizing it, remember you are erasing all information, thoughts, beliefs, and emotions related to this food and that you, yourself, attach to it.

In your other hand, imagine holding the problem that you wish to erase, or the food you wish to neutralize and make positive. In neutralizing it, remember you are erasing all information, thoughts, beliefs, and emotions related to this food and that you, yourself, attach to it.

Now hold your two hands about hip width apart and allow your palms to face one another. Notice there is a tension between your two hands. If you are used to feeling energy, you will feel it more strongly. If you are not used to feeling energy, you may feel a slight something, but not much. Perhaps you feel a tingling, hot or cold. It does not matter either way. Just trust it to happen. Do not try to make it happen, just allow it to. Notice how your hands feel as though they are pushing away from each other, as though there is a slight tension pushing them apart.

Now hold this position until the hands of their own accord begin to come together. It normally takes about a minute, sometimes slightly longer depending on what needs to be erased. In doing this, what you are actually doing is neutralizing and erasing all the information in this food, known and unknown to you. You are unifying and uniting all of this information with the hand that represents divine perfection. As the hands eventually come together the food will be transformed into the same energy of love—into the energy of divine wholeness, divine perfection, oneness, one power, one energy—and be free of polarity thinking. There is new information you are now putting into this food. You are giving it new power. You are deleting negative information, and increasing all the life-giving things about this food. You are making it pure perfect frequency.

Pay attention to how food feels before and after doing this exercise. You can even feel the vibration of the food before and after this exercise if you feel confident to do so. If you are right-handed, use your left hand to feel the energy. If you are left-handed, use your right hand to sense the energy. Hold your hand slightly away from the food without touching it, palm facing toward it. Notice what you feel. You might feel a sensation of heat, cold, tingling, or some other funny feeling that is there but is difficult to describe. Feel the difference before and after this exercise. This process may appear too simple, but do not be deceived by its simplicity.

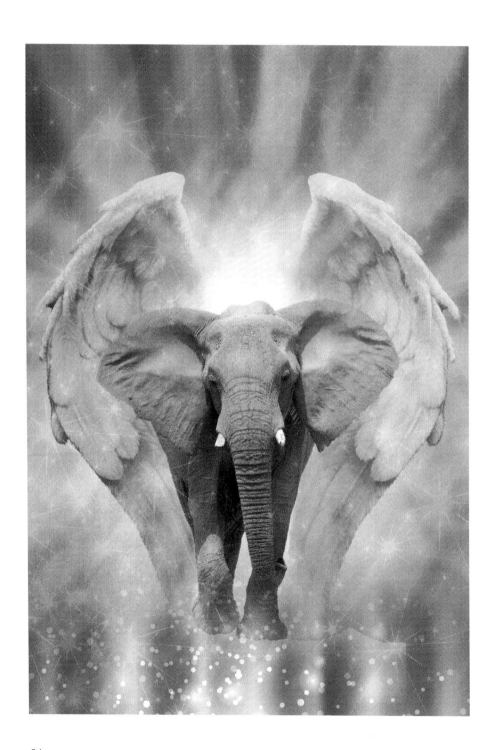

CHAPTER 6

EAT WHAT YOU LIKE AND STILL LOSE WEIGHT

Food, glorious food. The truth is everyone loves to eat. Food is a joy, a pleasure. You eat to bond with others. You eat when you are in love. You eat to celebrate happy occasions. Yet so much of the time what you put into your mouth is accompanied with guilt and a belief that you will be punished for this through weight gain. However, this weight is really only the result of your faulty beliefs. Beliefs that may include: I am never good enough; I am not free to feel what I really feel; I have no willpower; it's bad to be selfish; I need to be loved and approved of by others; I need to look perfect; and so on and so forth. You get the picture. What an important filter your beliefs form, both for the life you end up manifesting and for the body you wake up with every morning.

Your body only ever follows the filters of your many misguided beliefs, developed through childhood, your parent's relationships with their bodies and food, and a society obsessed with being thin at any cost. In fact you live in a society that is obsessed with image, and bases their innate value on the external body first, rather than the internal 'I.' Most people walk around in either food phobia or food guilt. You will either be someone who has given up on looking great, or be obsessed with bringing it about at any cost. Imagine if instead you adopted a new resourceful belief, such as, *"The more I eat the thinner I am."* What if changing your body was literally that easy?

Much of the time you may explain your body shape and size away on your genes, however, in his new book, *The Biology of Belief,* Bruce Lipton talks about the new science of Epigenetics, which literally means "control above the genes." Dr. Lipton explains that "Epigenetics is the science of how environmental signals select, modify, and regulate gene activity. This new awareness reveals that our genes are constantly being remodeled in response to life experiences. Which again emphasizes that our perceptions of life shape our biology."

Belief can affect outcome! Dr. Lipton reveals through various scientific experiments that orders from the mind can override the body's natural mechanism.

Dr. Lipton illustrates through the story of a boy healed by the power of the mind from a genetic disorder that "the mind can override genetic programming."

When your body gains weight, the first place you look for an explanation tends to be in the realm of problems, that is, you look to see what went wrong. Perhaps the first thing you analyze is your inferior behavior, such as eating too much or eating the wrong kind of food. You may also blame a physical imbalance, such as a slow metabolism, hypothyroidism, hormonal issues, and blood sugar imbalances. What is often left out of the picture is the role that thoughts, beliefs, and emotions have on the body, and in particular, in the creation of fat. Fat is an insulator, a protection. In my experience of working with people, I have never met an overweight person who is completely happy, in the perfect place in their life, has had a joyous upbringing, and is in complete inner peace. No, instead the overweight people I have come across tend to have huge inner turmoil, may have resentments they need to work through, have trouble being aware of their feelings, and often have limiting beliefs about themselves or life in general. In addition to this, however, the thin people I have seen over the years who are obsessed with being thin at any cost are like overweight people in disguise. They share the same emotional characteristics but just express them differently.

Have all the people I have treated over the past fifteen years been overeaters? Some have, but many have not. Is it therefore possible that unbalanced behaviors and health conditions that are seen as the culprits causing weight gain stem from somewhere else? Why is it that you have food behavior issues in the first place, and someone else does not? The key is to consider the role that your emotions, beliefs, and thoughts play in the creation of what appears on the surface to be the real problem, but may not be at all.

When you experience a significant emotional stress in the mind and body, your fight-or-flight response is triggered. This is a vital ability your body still performs, left over from the cave days, when you literally had to either flee from a wild animal coming at you, or stay to fight. Adrenaline pumps through your body and raises cortisol levels. As the adrenal glands begin to work in the place of normal energy, they often run out of energy very quickly, and can trigger weight gain, even if you are eating perfectly and exercising well. This is particularly true if your adrenal glands are taxed every day with high physical or emotional stress.

It makes sense that when we put the body into a state of weight loss, which is also a form of emotional and physical stress, we are faced with an interesting dilemma. If stress is the very thing that stops weight loss, and triggers fat gain, and weight loss itself is a form of stress, then how can someone succeed in losing weight? You can if you just continually stress the body more and more, where it has no choice, through tougher workouts or lower calories. However when the body is tricked into losing weight through overly stressful events, it will always have the last say, triggering the reverse and eventually gaining the weight back when the stress is over. The stress itself is putting the body into a cycle of wanting to put on fat again for protection. This is therefore not the best approach for long-term weight loss and longevity in general.

Limiting your food intake creates stress in the body, particularly if the intent is a limit of food for the sake of weight loss. Why? Because your body is an intelligent vehicle. It has a very deep and knowledgeable intelligence linked into a higher energetic one, and can tell when you are trying to change it forcefully, and particularly through lack of love. When you force your body to change because you reject it for how it is, in the here and now, it will rebel against you. On the other hand, when you naturally eat less or eat differently from a place of love, the body believes it is in a perfect state and acts accordingly.

The point is, your body can lose weight without stress, without any negative side effects to your adrenal glands, thyroid, or to other major glands in the body that are responsible for important hormone production related to appetite, metabolism, and physical health. Your body can lose weight this new and easier way. In fact it loses weight much better when it is in a complete state of equilibrium and harmony. This form of weight loss is very different than the one you may be used to hearing about. You may have been taught to stress the body both through intense exercise and through limiting food intake in some way. *"Do you want to lose weight?"* experts ask. *"Then you must cut out certain foods."* This is a very strong societal belief. Weight is all about calories in and calories out. Thus certain foods are considered ideal for weight loss and others not so good. At this moment in time the trend is to eat high protein and little or no carbohydrates. Perhaps this way of eating does produce results in weight loss, but at what cost? What is the ultimate effect that this is having on the body at a cellular level? You will find that this, too, stresses the body, requiring extra food intake after long periods of time and even potentially triggering binge eating. What will be the repercussions in ten to twenty years of following such excessive eating practices? Why do it this way, when it may not be the most agreeable way for your body, nor the healthiest long term?

Now, let me return to the assumption that your body is a living, breathing organism that reflects your consciousness. Your innate body intelligence knows what is best for it at all times. Let me give you an example. At one of the workshops I was running on this material, we were all neutralizing the effects of all the food—creating the food to be positive, healing, and energizing.

Then we each took a turn to ask, *"What food in this moment of time will bring my body into perfect equilibrium, perfect balance, and perfect health? What does my body want to eat right now for my highest good?"*

When I asked this, I heard my body clearly say to me "chocolate cookie." At the time of running this workshop I was having negative reactions to eating dairy (this is no longer the case, may I add), so eating a chocolate cookie was not allowed. Plus, at the time there was a residual belief in me that "this is not a healthy choice." But what if the chocolate cookie was precisely what I needed at that moment? What if it was going to help my body learn how to deal with dairy a little at a time? What if I needed the magnesium from the chocolate on this occasion? My body intelligence certainly seemed to think it was perfect for me. I didn't listen and did not eat it. I ignored my body's inner wisdom. When everyone went home for the day I knew I needed to eat the cookie, as the nagging feeling just wouldn't leave me. I gave in, ate the chocolate cookie, and felt great! I experienced no negative reaction whatsoever to having eaten it and from that day forth continued to eat dairy when I was naturally led to do so.

I spoke earlier of neutralizing the effects of food and this still holds true. All that is done through this book has an accumulative effect on your body, mind, and consciousness. The work you have put in so far is already producing the results. Now you are simply going one step further. Now you do not just want to stay the same weight, eating anything you want. Now you want to be able to actually lose weight at will. However willpower alone cannot produce the results that you seek. Listening to the deeper knowing of your body is also crucial. This deeper knowing and body intelligence knows precisely what your body requires to eat at any given moment. The question that needs to be asked from moment to moment in this state of perfect consciousness is therefore:

"What food at this moment in time contributes to MY perfect equilibrium, perfect balance, perfect health, perfect wholeness, and MY perfect weight?"

Put another way, *"Does this food lead me toward these things or away from them?"* So you are asking if this food moves you toward your perfect state of health, or away from it. Now you may think this is not much different from any other diet, but remember the answers you receive may not always be what you think. Sometimes to lose weight what your body needs is fat, sugar, or salt, and at other times it requires lighter food, but the point is you must ask this question each and every time, and you are asking about much more than just weight.

Remember you are neutralizing the effect of all food and in its neutral state, once you have done this, you are then asking the question. Now, just because all food is neutral, does not mean you are a garbage bin. You do not need to throw everything in yourself, even though you do not really want to. *"Well, I can eat anything, so I may as well do so."* No! Given you are free to eat anything you please, you can ask freely what you truly desire to eat. When you ask this question, it is not only about your body, your mind, your appetite, your hormones, adrenal glands, thyroid, metabolism—it is about everything. This question crosses the lines and boundaries of your whole being. It includes energetic aspects of yourself, informational aspects, and everything in between, across dimensions and across time and space.

"Does this food move me toward my equilibrium or away from it?"

This is the only question required. To make it easier for myself and my children, we simply ask, *"Is it a thumbs-up or a thumbs-down food for me right now?"* Easy! Or you can ask, *"Which food is good, better, and best for me right now?"*

How will you be able to hear or know the answer once you have asked? It may be difficult at first, with so much conditioning to wade through and too much knowledge about food that you have accrued over the years. But as you practice this consistently you will gain enormous confidence in hearing and knowing the answer each and every time. Practice is the key coupled with little or no attachment to what the answer will be.

However, this is not the end of it. The next step is CRUCIAL in being able to lose weight while eating anything you want. Let's pretend for a moment you asked the question about eating a giant piece of cake, and the answer you receive is that eating it at this moment will move you away from health, rather than toward (i.e., a thumbs down). But you go ahead and eat it anyway? Does this mean that you will now gain weight? Not necessarily. So long as you ask again when it is next time to eat, your body will choose a food that will balance you again. Remember you can balance everything! Everything can be brought back to Divine Being. All things can be realigned, unified, and corrected back to a love-filled place within you.

So sometimes you may get the answer that a particular food moves you away from health, but you know what, boy do you want to eat it, and you haven't had chocolate cake in years, so you eat it. But you eat it GUILT FREE. This is so vitally important to losing weight. You cannot imagine until you experience this in practice how powerful it is.

Eat it and be free of guilt.

The clarity and honesty of knowing that you are eating a food right at this moment in time that is moving you away from your equilibrium is what counts— the honesty. When you are aware of this, you do your body no harm nor cause it to gain weight, and it will come back into balance the next time around. Likewise, you can do this in regard to eating the correct quantity of food. When you are free of the restraints of negative emotions, such as guilt around food, this is pure freedom. Most people punish themselves for what they believe was bad behavior and even for having bad thoughts. No need for self-punishment again. Punishment never has been and never will be the way to motivate you forward. As Geneen Roth, in her book *Women, Food and God*, states, "When you abuse yourself (by taunting or threatening yourself) you become a bruised human being, no matter how much you weigh. Once you take the first few steps, once you begin treating yourself with the kindness that you believe only thin or perfect people deserve, you can't help but discover that love didn't abandon you after all." Only treating yourself with self-love will set you free once and for all.

Even though you may not have listened to your body intelligence on occasion, for whatever reason, the difference is you are doing it free from guilt. You are doing it with full awareness, and you have understood you do not need to be punished for breaking the good-eating rules. There are no rules. You are erasing all old rules that no longer serve you. You are coming back into your individuality, listening to the wisdom of your body. And if you choose to ignore its wisdom, then you are not punished for it, but loved and forgiven.

You are free to choose.

I am showing you a way to finally create your own system of rules. A system that is full of love, that you can trust and you always have faith in. It will never let you down. As you go through this shift in how you perceive food, you stop looking at your body in an accountable way, making sure it has done what you wanted. You stop checking it every second of every day either through scales or through what you wear. You stop judging it and looking for results. You begin to allow your body to naturally do what it does and you trust and have complete faith in it. Begin today to speak positively to your body. Say to it often that it is slim and well and say to yourself that it is effortless to be this way. What you believe to be true for your body, you create.

EXERCISE FOR CONSCIOUS CHANGE
TREE MEDITATION

Imagine walking through a park. A park filled with so many beautiful trees—big ones, small ones, tall ones, short ones, slender ones, thicker ones—and they are all unique. Each and every one is beautiful and wonderful just the way it is. You have no judgment of these trees, no view on a "good-looking" or "bad-looking" tree. You accept them all just as they are. They are all uniquely perfect. So too, each and every person is just as beautiful and each and every person deserves to be looked at like these trees—free from judgment, just allowing the beauty of who they are to be accepted and loved. So affirm right now . . .

"I release all judgment of myself and others about what I believe to be the perfect body. I release all judgment of myself as too fat or too thin, too tall, too short, fat bottom, protruding stomach, and big thighs. (Add in anything else you currently dislike). I forgive myself for being so hard on myself and expecting human perfection as set forth by someone else's standards. I am perfect right now and from this perfect place I now trust and step forward and do what is required for my perfect health. I listen to my body, trust myself, eat as I please, and always know the ideal thing for me to eat in every moment in time. I show only divine love for the self I was born to be."

Now imagine yourself surrounded by a beautiful golden light. Notice that it flows to you from above, and allow it to gently embrace you. Allow yourself to go higher and higher, higher and higher, higher and higher into the light. Keep going until you are in a place of great beauty, a special place just for you. Notice the landscape and the surroundings and know that you are safe here. In this sacred place you will see laid out before you a lavish banquet. Every food you could possibly imagine is on this table and you are free to eat anything, and as much as you want. All of these foods are presented to you and have already been neutralized on your behalf. They are all equal and produce the same effect on your body. They are all health-giving and life-giving, all at the highest possible vibration available. Just take a moment to ask, which food will bring you closer at this very moment to perfect equilibrium across all levels of your being?

Notice which food you gravitate toward in response to this question. Imagine eating it right now. Imagine chewing it, tasting it, swallowing it. Take your time. How do you feel?

Now, pick a food that you find moves you away from perfect equilibrium. Something that your consciousness and body don't really want to eat right now. Yes, all these foods are now equal, but for whatever reason this food is not right for you in this moment. Pick any food that feels as though it moves you away from your innate perfect health. Imagine picking it up and eating it anyway. Imagine eating it now. After you have eaten it, notice if there is any GUILT and allow the white light around you to take this ball of guilt away from you, every part of it. Make sure it has all been taken away. Allow any guilt from any part of your being—guilt from society's views about food; guilt from your childhood and the voices of others; guilt because you have now made yourself fatter or unhealthy; guilt that you didn't listen to what your body wanted; guilt because you believe you have no willpower— allow the beautiful light to melt it away, turning it into smoke and allowing it to evaporate. Now notice how you feel. Note that if you are too full your body still loves you. It will NOT go about gaining weight to punish you.

Notice that all you ever have to do to lose weight is to be in a calm, relaxed, and serene state. There is nothing in your life that can take this knowledge away from you now. Every time you eat, you will always be brought back to balance. Life is variable and sometimes you want to break your own body's rules without guilt. The good in you always draws you back. It is curiosity that occasionally rebels in you. Guilt is the greatest saboteur in life. It makes you a victim and pushes you to return to your fearful, child-like self. You can now be in a relationship with food where you trust it completely. You will never again fear food and its effect on you. You become empowered because now you are in charge of the food and what you eat, rather than being overwhelmed and controlled by it. Food is your resource and you can use it in a positive or negative way, as you choose to, without suffering any ill effects. When you truly believe this and know it unequivocally to be true, all stress around food will be removed from your life. Overeat? No problem. You will be brought back into balance on your next meal. You have nothing to fear and nothing to feel bad about and you need not suffer any negative consequences. Believe this and all stress will fall away. As it does, food will no longer trigger the fight-or-flight response in you. It will no longer engage your adrenal glands into battle and never again cause the ill effects that you believe made you overweight in the first place.

YOU ARE FREE!

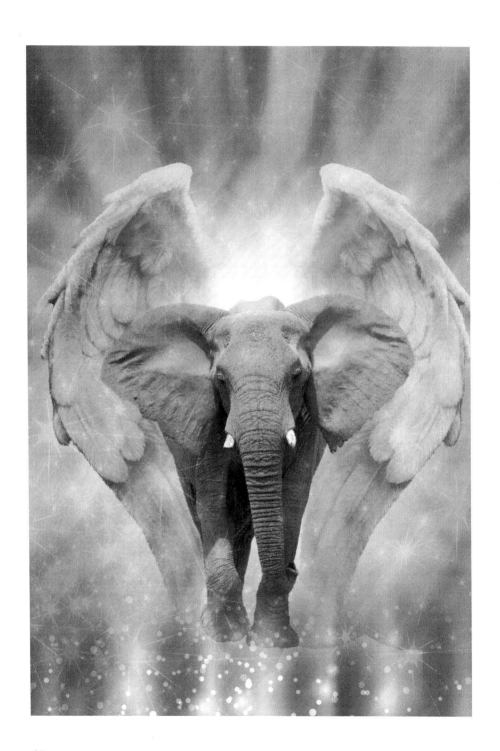

CHAPTER 7

DISCOVER THE JOY OF MOVEMENT

Your body is designed to move. Movement is a thing of grace and a thing of beauty. Movement of your body adds very much to your overall health and well-being. There is ample research that indicates good endorphins are released during exercise and contribute to mental and physical vitality. From the beginning of time it was imperative that you move. However, due to living a mostly inactive lifestyle compared to your hunter-gatherer ancestors, you now need to be more deliberate in your attempts to move your body. You need to build into your days, intentional movement whereas in times past, movement was just naturally part of carrying out the jobs of the day. Cars, computers, and television have all greatly impacted your attempts to keep your body moving. That being said, in this day and age where fitness and movement opportunities are plentiful, why is it that we move less than ever before?

Maintaining and enjoying a regular exercise program or movement endeavor depends largely on your reasons for exercising in the first place. Why are you doing this particular sport or movement form? What is your motivation behind it? Unfortunately many people exercise to avoid illness or death, to lose weight, or to gain the love and approval of others. Motivations such as these are extrinsic and largely fear based. Exercise based on these principles stems back to beliefs, such as, *"If I don't exercise I might get sick or FAT!" "I am not good enough the way I am." "I'm too fat." "I am unlovable as I am." "If I am slim then I am a more valuable person,"* and so on. Such beliefs fuel the current fitness industry rather than helping you reach inner peace and balance.

According to Sarah Grogan, in *Body Image: Understanding Body Dissatisfaction in Men, Women and Children*, "Women have always been encouraged to change their shape and weight to conform to current trends." Sarah Grogan says the motivation for women exercising, compared to men, is more highly related to weight loss. She describes how the latest research indicates that women and gay men are more likely to exercise in order to improve their appearance compared to heterosexual males. She also refers to research that indicates both males and females are now striving for more muscular bodies, hence they choose exercises accordingly. I was also a little alarmed at the potential for exercise to be used in harmful ways, when Sarah pointed out that exercise pressure is replacing diet pressure as the new way to stay slim. This is not how I envisage our ancestors using the gift of movement.

Allow me, if you will, to give you another perspective on movement and exercise. Human movement is a necessity because it keeps you feeling alive and positive. Regular body movement allows you to feel naturally good about yourself and to acknowledge and often discover your real and authentic self. Regular movement allows you to naturally release long-standing emotional blocks, to reach new heights in yourself, and to overcome internal challenges. Through regular movement you are offered the opportunity for a divine and magical energy to flow through you, and to feel naturally more connected to the universal mystery called life. It provides the opportunity for deeper self-growth, releases limited thinking, and improves every single area of your life.

The key to successful movement and exercise in a way that provides substantial results, I believe, is through doing something that is FUN. I do not believe in simply finding the most effective exercise to give you the results you want, if you hate doing it. Focusing only on the outcomes of exercise as the motivating factor will ultimately lead you to fail or give up. While having an outcome can be motivating for many people, when you move from a place of ambition (doing what you do for external reasons), to living life through deeper meaning and connection (doing what you do for internal reasons), you will reach higher outcomes than you thought possible. An outcome invented by your human mind will never be as tremendous or have as much potential as the outcome provided for you by a universe that will provide you with infinite energy and opportunities to play!

So when it comes to movement, keep it simple. Allow if you may your heart to lead and not your mind. Give everything a go until you find that thing or combination of things that brings you joy and makes you want to move, crave it even. The form of movement you choose needs to be something you yearn for. It needs to be something that you cannot wait to do again, not something you drag yourself to because you "should" or "have to" do. Beware of those words in your language. When you catch yourself saying them to yourself or to others, they are indicators you have slipped back into old rule-based ways of thinking that no longer serves you. Decide that you will bring joy to the movement that you choose, rather than expecting the movement to generate the joy for you. Be the creator of the joy, and the movement that you choose can then be the vessel for more joy to come to your body and to your life.

My focus in life is very spiritual, so I tried yoga several times because it is what spiritual people should be doing, but the truth is I really do not enjoy doing it. I'm not sure why. I just find it incredibly boring and uninspiring. My mind tried to convince me several times through statements like, *"What sort of spiritual person are you? You have to do yoga if you want to progress spiritually. Other people do it and you will not succeed without it."* Yes, I could have stuck with it anyway, but I listened to my own advice for a change and found something else I enjoy doing RIGHT NOW. Tomorrow I may love yoga genuinely and that's fine, but today it's just not for me.

Instead I love to participate in group circuit classes and love to do Qi Gong. These activities inspire me to willingly and excitedly jump out of bed every morning with vigor at 6:00 a.m., five days a week. I may not be the fittest, slimmest person in the world, but this is not important to me. I am, however, healthy, energetic, and enthused for the rest of my day when I do these exercises. They add quality to the rest of my life and they are joyful for me. Many people over the years have asked me how I am so dedicated in exercising the way I do. My answer? I do not have to exercise. Instead, I love to do it. Importantly, if I ever wake up feeling like it isn't right for me today, then I don't do it. I am not fanatical or attached to it. I do not live by rules when it comes to exercise and movement, but instead follow my intuition and my heart. Together they are rarely, if ever, wrong. How I look as a result of exercising is a side benefit for me. It is not what motivates me to move.

Synchronistically, just after I finished writing this chapter, I stumbled upon a movement approach known as Nia—Neuromuscular Integrative Action. I was flabbergasted to find that its first principle is called "The Joy of Movement," like the name of this chapter! Looking into this exercise technique more fully, I was amazed by its view of movement as something that needs to be guided by pleasure rather than pain. Debbie Rosas, one of the founders of Nia, says of exercise, "You can get fit and stay healthy by following the pleasure principle." Through changing the focus from exercising to look a certain way, to exercising to feel a certain way, Nia incorporates a fusion of dance, martial arts, and the healing arts together in its exercise classes. Movement is seen as medicine, and a way to tap into universal joy. Since participating in Nia classes, having discovered Nia only weeks ago, I am already tapping something deep within my feminine nature that regular exercise has failed to tap in me up until now.

You can tap into such a feeling, too, by following your own pleasure principle. Dedicate yourself to movement as a way of life. See it as something to bring you to life rather than recover from. I will speak of the importance of recovery later, but for now suffice it to say, Nia has been the only challenging exercise I have participated in where I did not need to undertake anything afterward to aid my recovery! To find out more about Nia I would highly recommend the book *The Nia Technique* by Debbie Rosas and Carlos Rosas.

So remember the key to moving is to find something that is highly enjoyable and fun for you. When it comes from this intent, you will find you lose weight and, even more important, gain health more easily than ever and love doing it. It will all happen when you are not even looking, because truly successful weight loss happens when you are just focused on having fun. You are already designed to move, so you cannot fail, just do not force yourself. Instead, allow yourself to flow to a movement that matches you today and makes you feel good. Challenge yourself, try different things until you find the right thing, and as a general guide, try something new at least three times to see if it really is for you or not.

Exercise and the challenge it sets for us physically can also represent a metaphor with how we deal with life's challenges. Those in the fitness industry have often thought that the tougher the challenge you can overcome in exercise, the tougher you are in dealing with life's challenges. If you can overcome what appears challenging in exercise, then you can overcome anything. While this is one way of looking at movement, what if through picking pleasurable exercise instead, you are saying to the universe that you are also choosing pleasure in life?

In regards to weight loss, many people do not realize that this occurs in between exercise, and not while you are actually exercising. Exercise itself is a form of stress on the body. So the wrong exercise and too much exercise can hinder progress with both weight loss and health improvements. The key to utilizing movement so that it works for you, in my experience, is correct and adequate

RECOVERY. This recovery needs to be physical and mental.

For me the power of Qi Gong is a powerful recovery system of health. It is highly beneficial for the recovery and strengthening of both mind and body. It rebalances the acupuncture meridian system which transports blood and chi throughout the entire body. I personally have a daily regime of some Qi Gong practice, as well as Qi Gong self-massage, which frees up blocked aspects of both the mind and body for full and speedy recovery. Proper recovery from movement is a fundamental step in the right direction for freeing up the energy of the body, releasing past limitations, and overcoming stagnant energy, in the form of fat, toxins, and organ dysfunction.

All of these methods as well as other forms of recovery such as massage, stretching, healing treatments, and just plain old rest also create movement in both the mind and body. All movement provides a cleaning and energizing action. Movement cleanses. It sends out old stagnant energy, making room for new energy to emerge.

I like to consider sleep a form of movement too. Sleep is highly beneficial and crucial for losing weight. Lack of sleep can very much hinder weight loss and health. The body needs to sleep well in order to recover fully. The body believes it is under stress and attack when it does not have adequate sleep time to recover and heal. It is in essence a form of movement because, even though you seem to be still, there is much internal movement that occurs. The movement of self-correction, self-healing, and self-regulating is happening and this is movement also. Not having enough sleep can create blockages in the body, just as lack of movement can.

Remember movement is beauty and it needs to be enjoyable and not be done just for the sake of it. You may also need to encourage yourself to try something different or you may never know that you will enjoy a particular activity. What about if you have a deep passion for tennis, golf, or surfing? Or you love aerobics, but do not consider these as options to try?

You may think these are beyond you because you feel so unfit, and they seem too hard to engage in. It may not feel enjoyable to begin with, but with time you will overcome the current mental and physical limitations allowing you to enjoy it from a deep place within you. Be kind to yourself and patient with your body. Stay with it while you give it a chance, and remember to do it for reasons of love and fun, and not do it merely to satisfy your external self. Anything that is done just to gain an external outcome can never last in the long term, and can even result in injuries. Movement is about joy and as long as it creates joy it will assist in all of your physical aims and in the accomplishment of all your physical dreams. It will also flood you with life and the joy of living.

Write a list of the activities you loved doing when you were younger in order to get an idea of what sort of movement you might enjoy participating in today. Generally, most kids still act from a place of internal motivation up until about age eleven or twelve. After this age, we tend to want to fit in, so we may join in activities to be accepted rather than because we like them. In your list be sure to add activities you loved to do, particularly around ages nine and ten. Are you surprised by what is on your list? Make a commitment to begin some form of movement practice in the next two weeks, just for you and just for fun.

EXERCISE TO ENHANCE PHYSICAL, MENTAL AND ENERGETIC RECOVERY AND BALANCE

This is an incredibly powerful exercise to balance you in so many ways. You will only know its amazing efficacy through experiencing it. It is just wonderful to do on a daily basis and need only take ten minutes a day. You will blossom in all ways from consistent practice.

Before you begin this exercise you will need to rest the tip of your tongue on your upper palate, where your teeth end and your palate or gums begin. Rest you tongue here for the duration of this whole exercise.

YIN YANG BALANCING TECHNIQUE

STEP 1: *Imagine a blue-colored light moving in the center of your body from the base of your spine to the top of your head, and down again. Imagine it pumping in this way, up and down, up and down. Notice if you can feel it, and if you can't just imagine it moving. Allow it to go as fast or slow as feels right. This is a cleansing and recovery exercise for the nervous system and spine. It also corrects the energy channels and communication from the spine to the organs and glands of the body. Do this for about a minute or until it feels done.*

STEP 2: *Breathe through your nose and allow the breath to fill your lower stomach, into what is known as the Lower Dan Tien, which is about three finger widths below your navel. Breathe out gently through your mouth. The dictionary meaning of calories is "units of heat," hence excess heat eaten in food can be easily released through the body and is actually released through the Lower Dan Tien area. This area also stores vital chi or energy for use by the rest of the body. Do as many rounds of deep breathing into this area as you like. Imagine a golden energy ball developing in this area. See it growing with every in breath and imagine it distributing energy and power to the rest of the body—including the internal organs, glands of the brain, muscles, and bones—on each out breath.*

STEP 3: *Imagine a golden light that begins in the center of the universe, pouring down and through the top of your head, through the center of your body, along the spinal column, and out through the base of your spine, into the center of the Earth, then emerging forward and up back into the center of the universe, and then back through the crown of your head again—all forming a circle. So it will be forming a circle that you are part of. Do this as many times as feels right, at your own pace. This step is very powerful at connecting you to your higher wisdom and grounding your true wisdom into the physical body.*

STEP 4: *Imagine a whirlwind of energy surrounding you. Give it any color or colors that feel right. Imagine this swirling energy, turning around your body in a clockwise direction, cleansing your aura of all energy and information you no longer need or require. It is also cleansing you of all stress that has accumulated throughout your day, as well as other people's energies that have impacted you.*

STEP 5: *Now imagine this same whirlwind of energy beginning to turn counterclockwise, cleansing old belief patterns and rebalancing thoughts and emotions throughout your being. Allow it to correct any information that needs altering and informs your body. Do this for as long as it feels right.*

STEP 6: *Imagine floating up as high as you can possibly go, to a place where there are no limitations and no illnesses or extra weight on you. Float to a place where you are totally well and complete, and just as you want to be in the here and now. Stay here for a while, until it just feels done and then imagine coming back down into your body. Imagine your feet being planted into the ground. Notice how you are feeling. Are you feeling wonderful, energized, and fully recovered?*

STEP 7: *Give gratitude and thanks for the gift that you have been given to create this miracle healing and balancing in yourself. You are the world's best healer for YOU! Give thanks to yourself. Make a commitment to do this every day. It is a powerful balancing exercise and is especially good at increasing your intuition and allowing you to bring through higher, more refined levels of creativity.*

CHAPTER 8
A NEW WAY OF BEING

What joy lies in your heart? What have you come to share with others? So long as you keep suppressing the wonderful gifts that you have to offer, your innate creativity, and the blessing of being who you really are, you will have difficulty dealing with your various emotions and will ultimately reach for food to pacify you. Food is your friend. It is now time to learn to be different in yourself and with yourself. It is time to learn to relate to yourself with great love, great compassion, great truth, and deep understanding. Do not see yourself as an imperfect being. No longer be so hard and judgmental toward yourself.

You are being granted, through this book, the freedom never again to be affected by food. It is not a matter of saying to yourself: *"I was doing so well and now I have failed and am falling behind."* You have understood somewhat that it is your beliefs that create your reactions to certain foods. It is now time to program your beliefs to be positive, to love to the highest vibration, so that you believe in yourself and find a new way of being within yourself and within the world. Your body is not something to fight against. Food is not something to fight. Weight gain is not something to fear. The world is not there to be fought with. All of these and more will support you when you begin to support yourself. When you begin to say to yourself, *"I am worth it. I do deserve to be on Earth. I have an importance and it comes not from what I do, but just from my being me."*

You are such a joyous wonder, a piece of the infinite, and a part of all things. You are a piece of the union of life and a vital piece of the universe. Therefore claim your power on this day. Understand that you can and are already beginning to place positive beliefs where negative ones stood before. You are beginning to believe that you are able to eat anything, as much as you wish, and never gain weight again, and indeed even lose weight. Claim your inner power and remove food as a causative factor in your life. It does not cause anything. Food is an effect, not a cause. All things are either a cause or an effect and food is an effect. It is the result of something. This something? This cause? Your thinking! Your thoughts are the only cause here. What you think and believe about yourself triggers powerful emotions, which then trigger stress. Are you thinking thoughts

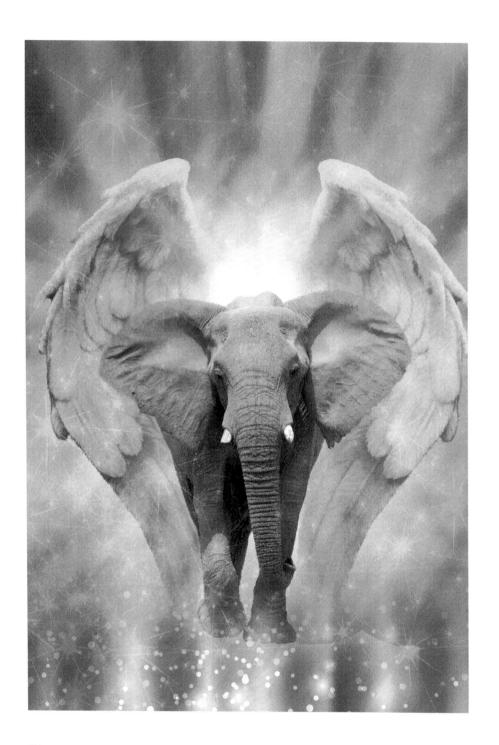

HELEN PAIGE

of love about yourself or are you thinking punishing thoughts? Are you thinking you are not good enough or not lovable?

Punish yourself no longer. Eat with joy and you will ultimately be drawn to healthy food. Of course, why wouldn't you be when you vibrate as you do and the purer the form of food the closer it is to the Divine Being? Natural food is always your first choice when you remove the limiting beliefs about yourself. The higher a food's innate energy, the more you are drawn to it. But this does not mean the times when you are drawn to other foods need affect you adversely. You will be so vibrationally clean and so vibrationally strong that nothing can ever hurt you again. Trust that this is happening now. Most of it has already begun. A good 55 to 60 percent is already in progress.

You will now continue on to explore your own eighty-one days of deep beliefs, emotions, thoughts, and behaviors relating to food, as you meander through my own experience of this to help inspire you. Each day you will read an entry from my journal, as I undertook this same journey myself, followed by the wisdom I received to correct my thinking and free myself from food. You will also find your own inner wisdom in the process. Through this you will find that the deepest part of your core, at the very cellular level, will alter. You will find your beliefs naturally change toward the positive flow and you will find greater meaning in yourself, greater meaning in your life, and greater meaning in food.

Sometimes the search for healing from food is the search for truth, inner understanding, and the search for your life path. Know that your path will be shown to you. You do not need to fear it any longer. You no longer need to suppress it or disbelieve by blocking it with food. Let yourself hear it and know it in the coming weeks, so that you may live your true life purpose. You are pure love, so allow yourself to be this love in all ways. Trust your body. Have faith in your body and it will finally support you. And you will finally be free.

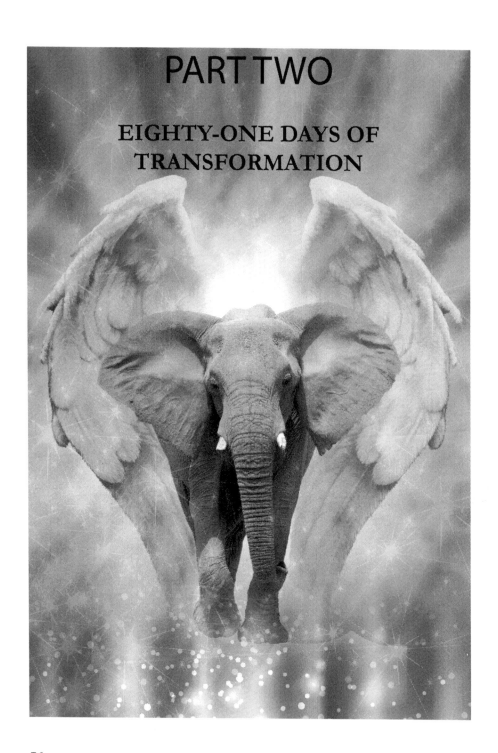

PART TWO

EIGHTY-ONE DAYS OF TRANSFORMATION

SWAP OLD "ELEPHANT BELIEFS" FOR NEW "ANGEL BELIEFS"

Congratulations on getting to this part of the book. You may need to reread Chapters 1–8 several times, when it feels right for you, to fully understand the many messages and learnings incorporated within.

You are now ready to journey through eighty-one old Elephant Beliefs and replace them with eighty-one new Angel Beliefs. Part 2 consists of eighty-one days of my own insights and learnings around food and my relationship to it. Read this as a path to change, and a way to help internalize the earlier part of the book. As you do this I encourage you to journal your own eighty-one days within which will change your own old Elephant Beliefs into new Angel Beliefs. In undergoing this process yourself, you are well and truly transforming yourself in relation to food. You will be able to eat anything you like and no longer gain weight. You will also be able to eat anything you like and lose weight!

Before beginning my own eighty-one days, I made the intention that I wanted to understand the deeper habits, patterns, and beliefs that I no longer required. In recognizing them, I understood the great power I gave to these beliefs and how they contributed to my body weight, my health, and my overall self-confidence. Understanding them not only helped me understand myself better, but also assisted me to understand what power I gave to food and how my thinking created food to be my enemy rather than my friend.

Why eighty-one days? There are eighty-one days in the *Tao Te Ching*, the ancient Chinese book of wisdom, authored by Lao-tzu. The *Tao Te Ching* and its eighty-one verses guide the reader through a path of inner transformation, and a way to live in peace, harmony, and love. Ultimately it is a path to changing your thoughts, and thereby changing your life.

The number eighty-one in Chinese philosophy is a yang or active number and comes together from 3 x 3 x 3 x 3 = 81. The number three represents creativity and is the last stage of creation.

The number eighty-one is also a result of 9 x 9 = 81, and eighty-one reduced to a single digit number equals the number nine (8 + 1 = 9). The number nine represents finality and completion. The number eighty-one therefore felt like the perfect number of days through which I (and now you) would change my relationship to food and my body forever.

Let me reiterate, you are about to read, in Part 2, my own recorded experiences and understandings over these eighty-one days. You will likely relate to most if not all of them, and learn a great deal more about yourself and your own limiting beliefs. As you undertake this, you are encouraged to undertake your own eighty-one days of transformation, where you will uncover even more thoughts that you pour into your food and your body. You can journal this in a notebook of your choice.

In addition you will find a "From Elephant to Angel Action" for you to do each day to further anchor these changes in yourself. If possible, it is also beneficial to undertake these eighty-one days with others who participate in this process with you. The support of others undergoing the same process is invaluable. This will add another dimension of encouragement and momentum to creating a whole new you. Then you will be well and truly on your way to *Eating Like an Elephant and Looking Like an Angel!*

DAY 1

Elephant Belief

IT IS BAD TO EAT ANYTHING OTHER THAN HEALTHY FOOD.

I have been so conditioned to think that I need to eat only healthy food day in and day out, and that I lack self-control if I cannot manage to do this. Now let's get real. How many people eat "perfectly" all of the time? Yet I am walking around believing I should be perfect, and since I am not, then to some extent I am a failure. Sometimes I can set such high and rigid expectations for myself, and then beat myself up for failing to meet them!

Today is about changing this old, outdated elephant belief into one of allowing myself to eat whatever I like. The aim is not, mentally, to ban any food, because when I do I only want that food more and begin to rebel against the voice of my body. Listening to the body less and less eventually leads to a disconnection from my body. I become disconnected from my intuitive voice, which tells me what I really need to eat, because I am always thinking about the foods I am not allowed to eat and judging myself when I eat them. Today I am learning a new approach to food, one that says I can eat anything I like, rather than believing I should only ever be eating what I consider to be "healthy" food. My body is intelligent. I only need to begin listening to it.

Angel Belief

IT IS SAFE TO EAT WHATEVER I WANT. ALL FOOD IS GOOD FOOD.

From Elephant to Angel Action

Do a Mind Map writing the word FOOD in the middle and then linking all the different things you associate with food all around it. Write down all the things that you relate to food, including your attitudes, current rules around food, current behaviors around food, and so on. Then say: *"I erase all these connections. None of them are real. Food is just food. All food is good food. Erase, erase, erase."*

DAY 2

Elephant Belief

I OVEREAT AT THE SAME TIME EVERY DAY, AND NO MATTER WHAT I TRY, I CANNOT STOP.

I am noticing that every day at the same time of day I am insatiably hungry and almost unable to stop myself from eating. No matter what I eat, or how much or little I am eating earlier in the day, I still feel this way every day at the exact same time and have been for a few months.

When I ask my inner intelligence, I am told that if I listen to my appetite I will uncover the true underlying messages of my appetite. When my life is in balance I will not feel like compulsively eating at the same time every day and instead will be set free to listen to a more natural desire to eat. My deepest self communicated the following Eating Clock as a guide to what my insatiable hunger or appetite is really saying about the deeper messages of my heart and soul. You may also find it of use.

Angel Belief

I UNDERSTAND THAT AN INSATIABLE NEED TO EAT AT A REGULAR TIME EVERY DAY IS REALLY A MESSAGE FROM MY DEEPER SELF. I LISTEN TO IT.

From Elephant to Angel Action

Spend at least seven days taking note of which time of the day you are most motivated to eat, even if you're not necessarily hungry, or the time when you tend to eat compulsively. Once you've identified the time which is most problematic for you, use the affirmation provided to begin to heal this from within.

THE EATING CLOCK

1 am/1 pm   I need to nurture myself, the individual, ME.

Affirmation: I make a vow to nurture myself, love myself, and meet all of my needs. I know that through doing this before giving to others, I have more energy, vitality, and love to give. *I am a priority in my life!*

2 am/2 pm   I need to spend time with loved ones. I feel alone.

Affirmation: I am never alone. I am always surrounded by love and support, first my own and then the support of others. I am making space in my life right now to spend more quality time with people that I love and love me. This is important to me right now and I honor this need in myself.

3 am/3 pm   I need to express my creativity and do something creative.

Affirmation: I am creative first and foremost. The very fact of my existence is such a brilliant act of divine creativity. I begin on this day to honor my innate creativity and to express it in ALL that I do. Every single thing that I do in my day is a sacred act of creation, and as I recognize this, I create with love and gratitude. *I am free to create!*

4 am/4 pm   I need to plan. I need to know where I am going in the future and how to get there.

Affirmation: I always know where I am going. I release all conflict in me today that confuses my mind and prevents me knowing what I really want for my life. I know what I really want, and always have done, deep down inside. As I trust myself to succeed in making my dreams a reality, I will reveal this to my conscious mind now. Knowing this, I am free to plan for the future which is mine to create. I know how to get there because my plan is a divine one and I have the support of the universe in fulfilling my Divine Life Mission.

5 am/5 pm	I need to balance all aspects of my life. I am feeling out of balance.
Affirmation:	Balance is inherently mine NOW. I allow myself on this day to embrace the inherent balance from within rather than from a mind full of *shoulds* and have *tos*. This is not real balance. True balance in my life is allowing myself to listen to and follow my inner urge in each and every moment. I honor my inner voice for it has wisdom and knowing. I am in perfect balance on this day and forever more.
6 am/6 pm	I have family issues that need to be resolved.
Affirmation:	The only family issue I have that needs to be resolved is an inner issue of not accepting that which is. My family is not against me. I recognize on this day that my family do the best they know how. As I now know better, I release them from all expectations and forgive them for not providing the love that I need. I now recognize that the only person who can love me as I require to be loved is me. I love my family and they love me and as I release all of our family issues today to the higher power within us, I know that we can be in harmony and peace with each other from this moment forth. I will now step forward in a relationship with my family based on acceptance and compassion. I will cease to take things personally as I understand that how they treat me is more of a reflection of how they feel about themselves and has nothing to do with me at all. I am free and I set them free on this day also.
7 am/7 pm	I am feeling blocked by life and feel I am not in control, but instead life is ruling me.
Affirmation:	Life is not blocking me. I am blocking me. In this realization, I relinquish all control that I have forcefully been trying to exert over my life and trust in a higher power within me to put all things right. I allow inner peace to be my

focus now, as I release all blocks within me that stop me from living this peace each and every day. Life cannot rule me. My thoughts rule me. I claim positivity, love, and only good to infuse my thoughts from this day forward and know my path in life is clear, strong, and full of wonderful adventures. I am excited to be living life and look forward to the exciting manifestations that I create to come to fruition. Life is good!

8 am/8 pm   I am questioning my self-worth. Money, ego, power, judgment—these are the things I am trying to break free from to gain internal peace.

Affirmation: I do not need to break free from my addiction to money, ego, power, and judgment. I only need recognize my addiction to these things. Through this recognition they already begin to lose their importance and begin to fade away as limiting forces in my life. I claim the good in these things, for there is good in all things. As I change my perspective I make space for love, serenity, and confidence in myself to come forward. I begin to trust life and the process of life, and as I do I begin little by little, day by day to see that I am a lovable, kind, and worthwhile person. I give gratitude for the person that I am and my self-worth soars. In doing these acts, I now attract others into my life that see only the good in me.

9 am/9 pm   I feel a strong desire to be of service and help others but my life situation at this time limits this.

Affirmation: I understand in order to be of service to others, I first and foremost need to value myself. I have value and am fulfilling my purpose just by being here. This is service enough for now. As I recognize this, I begin to acknowledge myself for being of service in so many ways I didn't recognize in myself before, from thinking good of others, to being there to listen to a friend. It is virtually impossible to not be of service. In my recognition of this, the universe now sends me more opportunities to serve in ways that enhance my life even more. Thank you!

10 am/10 pm   I feel a lack of confidence. I know that if I had more confidence, all else would be well. I need to learn to believe and trust in myself consistently.

Affirmation: Confidence comes from a place within, and not from having achieved in the external world or from the approval of others. When I focus on this as the truth, I begin to create an inner confidence based on believing in myself. I am a creative, imaginative, and inspirational being just having been born. I don't need to be good at something to have confidence in myself. I allow on this day my inner confidence to well over, and as I do I empower others to do the same. I vow to remind myself on days when my confidence appears to be low or missing, it is still here and I will look past self-doubt to rediscover it again.

11 am/11 pm   I want to change my life or aspects of it and I don't know how.

Affirmation: Change is easy. Change will come forward to claim me when I allow it to with sweet surrender, trust, and faith. Change is a natural part of life. When I stop trying to force change or avoid it, change happens effortlessly, especially when I am not looking or paying attention. On this day, I hand the responsibility for the change I so desire to the Divine All-knowing Being within myself, and claim that which now comes to me effortlessly in life. It is mine to be enjoyed.

12 am/12 pm   I don't yet feel full love and acceptance of myself. I don't think I ever really have and I don't know how to. I need to change my fundamental view of myself from a negative perspective to a positive one.

Affirmation: Love is not simply something that can be felt for myself but must be lived within myself. I will realize this completely and utterly when I recognize that the love I give to others and seek is a mirror to the deepest love that I have for myself. Because I live life giving so much love, I receive love for myself naturally through the giving. To fully love and accept myself, therefore, all that I need to do is remember who I really am, give gratitude for this each day, and continue to shine in the many ways that I do. I will be my own unique, authentic self and, in doing this, am living and expressing love always.

DAY 3

Elephant Belief

I OVEREAT AT EVERY MEAL AND THIS IS MAKING ME OVERWEIGHT.

First of all, I recognize that overeating is not technically a problem in this weight-loss approach, because as I alter the consciousness of my body to no longer gain weight, it won't matter how much I eat. However, I also recognize that overeating is generally not what my body or mind want to do most of the time and overeating may be having a negative impact on my health.

My body is designed to stop eating at a certain point, as it knows when it is full, and I can eat again when I'm hungry. I believe I don't overeat because I cannot stop eating and lack self-control. I believe I overeat and make poor food choices when I want to punish myself for failing in life, or to feel good in some small way through food. Yet, ironically, when I do this, the person I punish in protest is myself.

Many people might argue that changing the body to be able to eat any food without gaining weight is giving obese people permission to keep overeating, but I don't believe they eat these foods because they like them, or feel good as a result. Instead, I think they unconsciously eat them because they feel bad about themselves, think they are not good enough to be thin, or don't know how to treat their bodies with love and respect.

Being able to eat whatever I want and not gain weight means that food stops being my way of showing myself love or hate—food just becomes food. It has no meaning other than nutrients and the joy of food itself. With this understanding, food can stop replacing the joy of life and the anxiety of life. Food just becomes food. How wonderful to be able to eat anything I like and never again gain weight and even be able lose weight.

I need to trust that embarking on this journey will not create an out of control feeding frenzy in me every day of the week. Instead, it will create someone who lives life to the fullest, enjoying all that life has to offer, and eats when they're hungry in order to have energy and vitality to live life.

I find that as I shift to this new way of being that I stop or at least greatly limit the use of food as an abuse toward myself. Instead I look at what's happening in my life square in the face and feel what I feel completely without fight or flight. I find that I make lots of wonderful food choices because my new barometer is not my weight or self-punishment or reward, but instead it is acknowledging myself and feeding myself what really makes my body and mind feel good. All of me is coherent. I feel good, my body feels good, my mind feels good, and my emotions feel good, because they are being heard and acknowledged. I have found that little by little I have grown more sensitive to hearing what my body really wants to eat, and I serve it well rather than punishing it.

Today, my task is to pay attention to when I purposefully eat food that at this very moment in time, I still believe deep down, is going to make me fat, and to STOP just for a moment. In this moment I will instead ask myself:

"What am I punishing myself for?"

At the end of the day I will take some time to reflect how many times today I ate for self-punishment, or because I felt I was not good enough. I will state out loud, *"I am free to feel what I feel about myself—all of it. I do not need to hide how I feel about myself. Through knowing, I fully acknowledge myself and my feelings. I have value and worth and I am not a garbage bin to throw food away in. My body, mind, and soul are coherent and precious and I am now in the full process of separating what I eat from how I feel about myself or others. I am making wonderful progress and I believe in myself."*

Angel Belief

I AM FREE TO EAT AS MUCH AS I LIKE AT ALL TIMES AND AM SAFE TO DO SO WITHOUT GAINING WEIGHT.

From Elephant to Angel Action

Pay attention how many times today you eat what you eat, and still believe the food choice is bad for you. Recognize that through eating it anyway, you are choosing to punish yourself. Remind yourself that you are only love, forgive yourself for all that you think, and ask that "right mind" be restored in you, allowing you to eat with love and joy any food you choose.

DAY 4

Elephant Belief

I MUST NEVER EAT FOR THE WRONG REASONS SUCH AS TO AVOID MY FEELINGS.

Rather than spend the rest of my life in "inquiry" every time I eat, I will just eat when I eat, and won't when I don't. I don't want or see the need to eat "perfectly" all the time, such as eating only when I'm hungry, eating only when I'm sitting down, and certainly never eating when I'm feeling sad or angry. And if I commit any of these food sins, then it must mean there is something wrong with me and I will most certainly gain weight!

I'm what you would consider a very healthy eater, but I have days when I eat heaps of sugar, crunchy snacks, and white carbohydrates. Sure, sometimes I do this because I'm feeling anxious, overwhelmed, because I don't know what I'm really feeling, or just because it's my time of the month. This is life and so long as I'm an emotional creature, food will continue to be what I lean on sometimes.

Now, the difference as to whether the food that I have eaten will turn into fat or not is whether I believe I am safe or not. I remind myself that food is neutral energy and no matter what or how much I eat it ought not really matter.

I remind myself that if I overeat or eat for the wrong reasons, there is nothing wrong with me and nothing to fix. When I remind myself of this I return to eating healthier food. I believe more natural and highly nutritious food is more attractive to me than nutritionally empty food. When I am kind and forgiving to myself I revert back to eating such food again, without force or coercion.

Today I let myself off the hook for not eating perfectly. I will be kind and forgiving to myself when I use food as a substitute for not feeling all that I feel.

Angel Belief

WHEN I USE FOOD TO AVOID MY FEELINGS I AM FORGIVING TO MYSELF AND AS A RESULT I DO NOT GAIN WEIGHT.

From Elephant to Angel Action

Today notice when you are not eating perfectly. Perhaps you are standing up and eating? Perhaps you are eating on the run, or eating something because you had a really bad day? Forgive yourself as you notice. Now that you have noticed, what do you really want to eat instead? You won't get fat either way, but now you get to choose from a conscious place.

DAY 5

Elephant Belief

I CAN'T EAT ANYTHING I WANT AND STAY THIN.

There is something in my consciousness that believes I can't eat anything I want and still be thin, especially given I am female. Men can, but I can't. Of course translating this belief to my entire life, does it also mean I can't have everything I want in life? Do I believe that I need to first ensure that my children, husband, and everyone else is happy—then me?

I pretend to look after myself through buying nice clothes, makeup, and pampering treatments, but the truth is I still often feel like a slave to others. Was I born to serve? As a women, am I loved for my compliance and ability to love and look after others? I believe it is time for this to shift in me. It is time for me to take accountability and responsibility for myself. It is my highest priority to find and live my joy. Let me emphasize here, it's not about finding my purpose. Usually a purpose is about asking *"What am I here to do?"* or *"How may I serve?"* Joy need not be about service. In fact joy is more likely to be accessed through the moments of just being—where I don't have to do anything to be loved, accepted, and worthwhile. When I access these moments, I actually become a divine channel of inspiration. The last time I went on a being phase and a sabbatical from doing, I was a phenomenally fully present mother and I developed and recorded a new healing CD all within a month. People think being phases are lazy, unproductive periods, but instead they are creative, inspirational, real, connected, and divine spaces. They are spaces where we can just be our true authentic selves.

When I flow with authenticity I allow my true essence and creativity to flow through me and quite simply, I create magic. I believe I am on Earth to learn how to be in the being phase permanently, 100 percent of the time. The truth is I don't really need to learn this—I came knowing, but I was taught that through doing I would become somebody that matters, somebody that's important. So I joined the tribe in order to fit in, be loved and approved of, and started looking for something to do. Deeply unsatisfied with this I now look for deeper meaning in my life—the secret jewel that can transform my mundane life into an extraordinary life and find my way back to being. Translating all this back to food—I can eat anything I want just like I can have anything I want from life!

Today I will write a list of all the things I would love to do, have, and be, just for me. I find it helpful to do it the way recommended in the book *Five Wishes* by Gay Hendricks. It's a great read.

I imagine I am lying on my deathbed and someone asks me, *"Has your life been a complete success?"* Assuming I answer no, I then proceed to list out why. *"My life was* **not** *a complete success because . . . "* Asking this question in this context triggers my mind to think of the things that really matter to me.

I did a fasting technique once for six days, where I was required to not eat or drink any real food or water, and instead I had to imagine eating all day long as though I really was. Using only my imagination I was allowed to eat anything I liked. What a great technique to show me what I really wanted to eat, but normally wouldn't have allowed myself to. I was eating scones, lasagna, hamburgers, salad, and fruit too! I was so surprised by some of my food choices. It highlighted to me that, perhaps, I don't always eat what I really want. Perhaps I am equally dishonest about what I really want in my life too.

Angel Belief

I CAN EAT ANYTHING I WANT AND STAY THIN FOREVER AND I AM EQUALLY FREE TO HAVE ANYTHING I WANT IN MY LIFE.

From Elephant to Angel Action

Using Gay Hendricks's technique, imagine you are on your deathbed and ask yourself *"Has my life been a complete success?"* Proceed to list out why either yes, it was or no, it wasn't. For example, *"My life was not a complete success because . . . "*

Once you have a list, then change these statements to the positive format. For example, *"My life was a complete success because I finished writing this book"* and so on.

Now write a list of *"If I could eat anything I wanted without gaining weight I would love to eat . . . "* What a great exercise for revealing the truth to yourself.

DAY 6

Elephant Belief

MY BODY IS NOT GOOD ENOUGH THE WAY IT IS.

I think I love to WANT things. I'm addicted to it, just like I'm sometimes addicted to conflict. I think this energizes me and makes me feel alive. Every woman I have ever spoken to has a part of her body she is not satisfied with and would love to change. Even the naturally skinny, super-sexy ones still are not completely satisfied with themselves.

I'm sure I wasn't always like this—so dissatisfied with my body. I remember as a child thinking my body was beautiful and being rather proud of it. I reflect that my current perceptions of my body are really other people's perceptions, as well as society's beliefs about what sort of body is considered socially beautiful and what is not.

However from the place of satisfaction and acceptance, the seeds of very real and lasting change can take place. I believe I will have finally "arrived" in myself when I can look at another woman walking past me and not think, *I would love to have her legs.* Instead, wouldn't it be amazing to be totally grateful and satisfied with my own legs, just as they are? I believe that it is possible to be completely and utterly in love with my body just the way it is. I believe that the day will come when I will not want to swap it, not even for a more slender one. It's mine. It's unique and it's wonderful in every way. Having longer, more slender legs, for example, will not make me any better. Only fully accepting myself can make me better.

Perhaps I believe I would have more power if I had what I consider the perfect body. Sure I remember having a flat stomach and a voluptuous bust in my youth and feeling very powerful—for all of five seconds. I was feeding on other people's opinions of me at the time, but they didn't even know the real me. Inside I felt more powerless and insecure than ever.

So today I will spend the day purposefully looking at other women who I consider as having more of a "perfect" body than me. As I do this throughout my day I will forgive myself for thinking other people's bodies are better than my own, by affirming in my mind *"My body is perfectly me!"*

MY BODY IS PERFECT JUST THE WAY IT IS. I LOVE IT RIGHT NOW AND ALWAYS WILL, NO MATTER WHAT SHAPE AND SIZE I AM.

From Elephant to Angel Action

Spend your day paying attention to what you are thinking about the bodies of other men or women you come across. What is it you envy or wish you could change about your body?

Right now, state the following affirmation:

"I accept my body as the perfect body for me right now. I release my need to look like others, and give thanks for the body that has housed me and looked after me all of my life. I am special, and that other person is special too. We are both unique and wonderful. I forgive myself for placing that other body above my own. I release my desire to want any other body than my own. I forgive myself for judging myself as imperfect. I love my body and accept it just the way it is for it houses my precious life force. It is me and I thank it and ask its forgiveness for all the times I have treated it badly. I am perfectly me right now. I have arrived in me and I accept myself fully."

DAY 7

REST DAY

Every seventh day is a day of rest and renewal in this process. This is a day where I will allow myself to give gratitude for all that I have, and to praise myself. Through doing this I will cultivate the soil in which my new Angel Beliefs are being planted. I will water these beliefs through self-praise and allow them to grow through gratitude for all the wonderful things I already have in my life.

Today I will praise my feet and ankles. I will spend the day feeling them more and thanking them for all they do for me.

Swollen ankles can relate to the following intuitive understanding:

Where am I walking to? Do I even know? Deep down I know what I want, and now is the time for me to finally allow myself to step into the life and future I have always dreamed of.

On this day of gratitude, I practice the acronym A.N.G.E.L as detailed in chapter 1 to change this for myself. You can do the same. Then write down a list of five actions you can commit to in order to get moving toward what you really want. Get back on your path.

DAY 8

Elephant Belief

EATING FOOD WITH TOO MANY CALORIES CAUSES ME TO GAIN WEIGHT.

Everyone is thinking about how many calories food has, but I think, how much love does this food have? To me the calories of food mean nothing, but the amount of love in it is the really important data. I want to allow food to give me its love and nurturing energy.

Today I make a pledge and promise to myself to never again be frightened of any food and its effects on my body. I just need to have faith in my body and trust it. It works for my highest good. It will look after me if I trust it. I have faith in the universal law that states any and all food eaten with love only nourishes me. This intent neutralizes all other negative information in food (including calories) and brings it back to being neutral. Then I can transform it to life-giving food. I cannot gain weight EVER from LOVE food. Today I make a pledge to love myself, trust myself, and have faith in my body! Calories are meaningless; only the percentage of love in food counts.

Food is my friend—all food—carrots and chocolate cookies are equal. I eat what I choose from within me because it feels right for me NOW. This is what I do now. I release all external influences and am fully present in myself. I listen. I trust. I AM.

Angel Belief

ALL FOOD IS LOVE FOOD. ALL FOOD!

From Elephant to Angel Action

Write a pledge to yourself like mine above, sign it and put it somewhere you can see it occasionally so that when the world tries to convince you of limiting beliefs again, you can read it and remind yourself of the true holistic and divine nature of all food. Also promise yourself to never read the calorie information on food labels. It isn't true. There should be a love percentage instead!

DAY 9

Elephant Belief

I NEED OTHER PEOPLE'S APPROVAL IN ORDER TO BELIEVE IN MYSELF.

I need no one's approval but my own. I live for me. I love me. I am not selfish but self-loving. I need to be of service to me first and only then to others. I have plenty to give to others when I am full. When I am full of my own self-love and self respect, I expect nothing in return from others in the form of love and approval for all that I give. I do not need to always love and approve of myself in order to give to myself. I can just give to myself and enjoy receiving.

The only person that ever really needed to believe in me was me. Yes, ME.

Why do I give more power to that one person that doesn't believe in me rather than to the many that do? What will it take to convince me? It's a choice really, and one that I can make right here, right now for me. I will state *"I believe in me. I am an amazing, incredible person with unique talents and abilities. I am me and no one else can be me, only I can, so from this moment forward I am being myself with gusto and passion!"*

I made a major error in my thinking based on my past. I believed the negative thinking and judgments of me made by others. Granted I was too young to know any better at the time, but now I am older and wiser. I know these people were not telling me what is true for me, but what they believed was true for them.

I can choose to reject this now. I know I can be nothing other than the good, the vibrant, and the alive presence that I am.

Do I need to be angry with, or pity, those people that lied to me? No, I need to send them love and compassion, so they can recognize that someone once lied to them too. Sending them compassion will break this chain of events from perpetuating further. Now I'm not only changing my past, but my future too, and my children's future! Today I sit and write a list of all the negative beliefs that people have provided me around food. Then I list all the judgments other people made about me that I adopted as my own. I burn this piece of paper and am free of them. Today I begin afresh.

Angel Belief

I NEED NO ONE ELSE'S APPROVAL IN ORDER TO LOVE AND APPROVE OF MYSELF. I BELIEVE IN MYSELF NOW. I AM FREE TO BE UNIQUELY ME!

From Elephant to Angel Action

State the following just like I did: *"I believe in me. I am an amazing, incredible person with unique talents and abilities. I am me and no one else can be me, only I can, so from this moment forward I am being myself with gusto and passion!"*

Create your own list of negative beliefs you have about food or your body that you KNOW have come from other people. These other people can be your parents, friends, relatives, experts, and anyone else you believed. Burn this piece of paper (safely), recognizing these beliefs are not really yours but other people's beliefs.

You are now free to adopt your own beliefs that better serve you. You are unique and one of a kind. Your new beliefs will be yours from the ground up. You are the creator of them, not others. Now begin a brand new list, and write the heading: My Beliefs About Food and My Body. Then begin writing three new beliefs that you have about food or your body, having read this book so far. You can add to this list naturally as you observe new beliefs emerging in you. You are on your way to creating a new way of seeing yourself and food.

DAY 10

Elephant Belief

I ALWAYS NEED TO BE DOING SOMETHING IN ORDER TO FEEL USEFUL AND VALID AS A PERSON.

I was thinking this morning that I would like to shift from eating lots of empty-type foods to eating more densely nourishing foods. In other words, I would like to eat less food, but better quality, rather than more food that is light and empty. Why is quantity so important to me? Why is the act of chewing something incessantly so appealing and necessary for me right now?

I think it's about always needing and craving to think. It feels like an attachment to love of thoughts, doing, and achieving, which are all active. Eating is active energy. However, active "doing" energy needs to be balanced with "being," which represents the act of digesting and assimilating information, energy, and food.

Eating anything so long as I'm eating is a bit like doing anything so long as I'm always busy, always distracted, always moving. To me it feels like I'm pretending to myself to be living and eating, but not being fully present in either.

On the other hand slowly eating nourishing food, with full awareness, is about quality of life. So eating in this way shows variety, depth, and nourishes my body deeply, just as I nourish my life and being by living this way.

I know my body will not begin to lose weight while I am not completely present and aligned in mind, body, and spirit. This may sound like a difficult place to get to in this hectic lifestyle that I live, but I know I can do it.

Being healthy means having healthy thoughts and beliefs about myself, others, and my life. It means eating in a high vibrational way, eating everything with an attitude of love, and genuinely believing that any food and all food is life-giving and life-enhancing. It means learning inner strength through the full expression of my emotions and feelings rather than suppressing them.

So my journal experience will not only transform my body so it no longer gains weight from food and loses weight if required, but it will transform who and how I am in the center of this thing called *my life*.

Through accepting each and every moment as a precious moment to "be in" first and foremost, then slowly my "doing" will also become filled with meaning and life-enhancing qualities.

Angel Belief

I AM FREE TO "BE" RATHER THAN ALWAYS HAVING TO "DO." AS I RELEASE THE NEED TO ALWAYS DO, I ALLOW MANY OF MY FALSE MOTIVATIONS TO FALL AWAY.

From Elephant to Angel Action

Make a regular time every day to do nothing. Nothing means nothing! Just sit quietly and be with yourself. Observe what is occurring around you. Notice what you notice. Allow yourself to unwind and relax during this time, and forget for a moment all the things you could be doing. Just be in the moment. Show gratitude for it and appreciation this is all you ever have to do to be loved and approved of. All the "doings" are just extra things you do. It is this "being" time that makes you. Begin initially by doing nothing and being for five minutes, and then slowly, as you are ready, expand this time to as much as an hour or longer.

I remember when I first started this practice it was virtually impossible for me to do. First I began by spending it thinking of all the things I would do once my time was up! I initially started doing this exercise when a practitioner told me that I would never find my true hidden passion in life unless I did this exercise. What motivation! I had to keep going. Not only did I discover it, but I also discovered me in the process. I have since come to learn that the art of doing nothing is just as important as all the active things that I do. I love it. With practice and patience, I know it will pay off for you too!

DAY 11

Elephant Belief

I DO NOT FEEL SAFE AROUND OTHER PEOPLE.

When I am working with clients I have this attitude that I never take what might normally appear offensive behavior of clients personally. Of course, they're rarely expressing the perfection of who they really are when they come to see me. All their human imperfections are being triggered by the intelligent universe in my presence so that I can help transform or eliminate them. My attitude allows my clients to return to their naturally healed states of being, which is who they really are in the first place. The limiting behaviors, attitudes, and beliefs in them are the result of life and other people conditioning them. My job is therefore to see the "real" them, the whole and perfect them, and return them to this light happy space, both energetically and physically.

I used to only do consultations one day a week. My personal challenge was to spread this attitude to the other days of my week when I was not working. During the week I would try to have this same attitude of not taking people's conditioned behaviors and imperfections personally and forgiving them, as I do on consultation days. After all, if I could do it sometimes, why couldn't I always think and act this way? I reasoned that this was because, during the week, I would go back to being conditioned Helen, with many buttons of my own that could be pressed.

When I began to transform this in my own life and, slowly but surely, made my attitude on working days spread through my whole week, it felt like I had lost so much energetic weight that was holding me back and weighing me down.

I also began to lose real weight that had been very resistant up until that point. This weight was my protection from what I perceived to be an unsafe world. As I realized that everyone is completely whole and well, vibrant and healed, my own buttons disappeared off me, just like they did on consultation days. I stopped taking other people and their behavior personally. I began remembering all through the week that people's behaviors, attitudes, and feelings toward me had nothing to do with me. Instead all it revealed was how they felt about themselves.

I remember hearing the spiritual teacher Eckhart Tolle asking in a talk, *"Would you be upset if the wind came along and destroyed your house versus another person coming along and destroying it?"* He pointed out that you wouldn't really resent the wind or want revenge, but of the person, you would want both. Yet the person is just as unconscious as the wind. They are not awakened to what they are doing or why. They are unconsciously acting toward you how they feel about themselves.

Hence as I now begin to see in all people, who they really are—beautiful light-filled, perfect Beings—I have stopped attracting people who treat me unkindly. I now attract people who show love and respect because these are the only qualities in people I pay attention to. I don't even notice anything else.

Angel Belief

I AM SAFE WITH ALL PEOPLE, AS AT THE CORE OF EVERYONE IS LOVE.
I TAKE NOTHING PERSONALLY, AS I KNOW THEIR BEHAVIOR HAS NOTHING TO DO WITH ME.

From Elephant to Angel Action

Spend the day noticing what behavior in other people upsets you. What are you taking personally? Notice this on the road as you are driving, even as you watch television, as well as in any interaction with other people. If you hear negative gossip, or find out that somebody doesn't like you, pay attention to how this makes you feel. Discovering how and where in your life you take things personally is a great way to bring your attention to the many times you make yourself upset for no good reason. Like the wind in the above example these people are only behaving this way because they lack higher awareness in this moment—it isn't personal even if it sometimes feels that way.

Decide today that you will begin a new way of being, where you cease to take anything personally. As you commit to this, pay attention to how others begin to treat you with more respect and love.

What sort of people do you now attract into your life?

DAY 12

Elephant Belief

WHEN I EAT FOOD THAT I BELIEVE
IS BAD FOR ME, IT HARMS MY BODY.

When I eat something on purpose that I believe is bad for me, then I am purposely trying to hurt myself. It doesn't really matter what the food is. I recognize that it is my intent that is making this food poisonous for my body and poisonous for my self-esteem. Why else would I eat something that I believe is bad for me? Of course, no food is bad, but because I think it is, I therefore make it poisonous for my body and health.

Today, as I was at the bakery, a lady being served said to the service attendant, *"Can I please have one of those pizza slices? Yes, the one that is really super fattening, please."* They were her exact words! Well, the attendant said back to her, *"I know it is so fattening, isn't it? You should have seen what I ate this weekend . . . "* You get the point. Well, guess what that food would have turned into when that lady ate it? It will have turned into the very thing she thought about it—FAT! I wondered, at the time, why someone would purposefully eat something that they fear will make them fat. This to me does not sound like being nice and loving to oneself.

I remind myself that I am a brilliant, perfect person, and all food is brilliant and perfect too. When I eat really knowing this about myself, food cannot harm or affect me. If, or when, I lack self-love, have self-judgment, guilt, shame, or believe I am undeserving, then I cause the food to create a negative response in my body and thereby trigger fat storage to protect me. No food is bad for me, only my beliefs about myself and the food I eat are bad for me. I will pay attention, too, when I decide to eat something I believe is really bad for me, and possibly make a better choice. Why point a bullet at myself on purpose? I'm worth more than that.

Angel Belief

ALL FOOD IS NEUTRAL.
I WILL NO LONGER PURPOSEFULLY
USE FOOD TO PUNISH MYSELF.

From Elephant to Angel Action

Today concentrate and dedicate yourself to only eating food that you believe is good for you. Write a list of the foods that you believe are not good for you, or which you think are fattening. Go through the list and focus on creating an intent that makes these foods neutral so you are allowed to eat them too. Until they have been neutralized, eating them will cause weight gain, so keep doing this exercise until you genuinely feel that all these foods on your list are just as friendly as the foods you already think are healthy.

Make this exercise even more effective by doing The Unification Process® you read earlier in the book and remember that all food is either "good, better or best."

DAY 13

Elephant Belief

I HAVE TO CONTROL MY EATING AND MY BODY IN ORDER TO STAY THIN OR LOSE WEIGHT.

The human body was not designed to be controlled. Nor was the human spirit. Most people hate being told what to do and hate being controlled by others. Yet this is what I do to my body all of the time. I try to force it to look a particular way, to act a particular way, and to be a particular way. Instead of succeeding, in the long term I end up imprisoning myself through too much control over how I live and eat, or I lose control all together.

Instead, I need to understand a crucial detail if I am to find the secret to weight loss without ever again needing to worry about what I eat. The body knows what it needs to do to be slim. Each person has a different point of slimness and this is not necessarily what the media would portray as slim. To be slim is to know that you may eat naturally, based on hunger and desire, and to know that your body will stay within its natural healthy weight range. This weight is different for everyone and it is probably slightly heavier than the "ideal" body portrayed by the media. My body has an inner intelligence built into it. It does not need me to decide and count calories or to eat tasteless food.

My body knows what to do. My body knows exactly how to bring me to health and wholeness and I must stop trying to force it. Through force I enter into a battle of wills and my body image suffers. I need to rise above control in order for my body to reach its natural self-sustaining level of slimness.

My body will never find this proper level through the notion of control, for control pushes me one way and then eventually my body fights back and pushes me back again. The same thing holds true for excessive exercise. The more I exercise the more I must keep exercising in order to continue losing weight or even maintain a certain weight. Likewise with food, if I reduce my food intake, then I need to keep reducing it even further in order to keep losing weight until eventually I'm hardly able to eat a thing!

A weight-loss approach based on control and force is therefore not for me.

This is not the ideal way in which to get my body and soul to work together.

My body ideally works in partnership with my deepest self. Both are equally important. I know that if my deepest self is not happy, my body will gain weight. When my body is not happy it will gain weight and my deepest self will also suffer and feel limited and resentful. They ought be a partnership. One cannot force the other. They need to work together to understand each other and to work as a team. I understand today that my body and deepest self, or spirit, need to be in alignment with each other for my optimal health.

Angel Belief

MY BODY DOES NOT REQUIRE ME TO CONTROL IT IN ORDER TO BE SLIM, HEALTHY AND FIT.

From Elephant to Angel Action

Write down a list of everything that you fear will happen if you relinquish control over your life, your body, and food. Look at this list and take a deep breath as you imagine handing these fears over to a higher power to take them away. Just imagine handing them into a bright white light that erases them. They are not real, but simply unfounded fears from the past. Look at your list again and notice how you feel about them now. Write next to each of your old fears, *"This is no longer true because . . . "* and state to yourself, *"There is something even better than control and that is freedom."*

As you relinquish a little more control each day, you will find miracles unfold in your life. Every time you become aware of controlling anything in your life, just close your eyes and hand it to the white light, just like you did with your fears.

This exercise will help you see the less in control you are the more easily your life flows. You will only believe me if you try it for yourself. Control is highly overrated!

DAY 14

REST DAY

Today I spend the day praising my legs. I look at the whole of my legs and praise all the great things about them. I especially praise my thighs. Truth is, I find it hard to love my thighs. I feel as if I have extra fat on my thighs that will simply not budge, and I remember that the metaphysical connection for this relates to fear of the future and a fear of success. I release these fears now through the A.N.G.E.L process.

I give gratitude today for all the opportunities that this day presents me with. I give gratitude for all the wonderful food choices I have today and gratitude that I am healthy, whole, and able to move and express myself as freely as I can. I look past any limitations that are bothering me today and focus on expanding the good that I have in my life and in my body. I give thanks to my legs for carrying me in life and being strong and healthy. I give thanks to them for taking me on wonderful walks through nature that I especially love.

DAY 15

Elephant Belief

I AM MOTIVATED TO LOSE WEIGHT THROUGH UNHAPPINESS AND JUDGMENT.

There have been many instances where I run out of steam when exercising. Exercising becomes a struggle and my body seems to go downhill with sore muscles in my neck, back, and all over.

On this particular morning, I realized the subtle error in my thinking that has been creating these occasional downhill slides in me. At those times, I realize my goal and my motivation suddenly becomes, *"I need to lose weight"* coupled with the even more subtle belief of, *"I'm ugly, fat, out of control, and not good enough."* These sorts of thoughts seem to sneak back in as a constant reminder that I couldn't possibly always love and accept myself as I am. There always needs to be something to change and improve in myself. It is as though I fear being happy and being self-content would make me too complacent and lazy, causing me to suddenly become even fatter!

Of course, when these episodes occur for me they are usually accompanied by the insatiable desire to eat everything in sight. When I want to punish myself for this lack of willpower, I will start thinking of all the potential diets I should undertake. With this decision, the last bit of self-love, self-acceptance, and self-trust goes out the door. No wonder during such times, I am hardly able to exercise at my best. There is no joy present and certainly no fun. Exercise becomes my version of the fat farm again!

Today I spend my day noticing the motivations behind all my actions. It will be interesting to see which of my motivations are related to self-judgment and harsh expectations of myself, and which ones come from a place of love and joy for myself and for life. I will do this activity in relation to what I eat as well as everything else in my day.

Angel Belief

I MOTIVATE MYSELF THROUGH LOVE AND SELF-ACCEPTANCE AND FORGIVE MYSELF FOR ANY JUDGMENTS ALONG THE WAY.

From Elephant to Angel Action

Today carry a piece of paper or notebook and pen with you. Notice when and how you are judging yourself through the day, and write these down. Review your list in the evening. First, acknowledge that no matter how true you feel these judgments to be, through self-judgment you will never grow to the next level of your wholeness. Forgive yourself for being so unkind and unloving to yourself.

Now look at your list again and scribble out any of them that you know are not really true. With the ones that remain, decide to use these judgments to motivate you into positive action rather than to limit you. Decide through self-love and patience to see these judgments not as condemnations, but as possible suggestions for improvement. This is called reframing, turning what seems negative into something positive to help you take positive action.

DAY 16

Elephant Belief

I AM POWERLESS TO RELEASE OR CHANGE MY CURRENT PERCEPTIONS.

In order to lose weight, and transform my body, I need to understand that everything is made up of information. Information from past, present, and future contributes to energy or matter, which then contributes to ME—my emotional, mental, and physical states. We are all the sum total of a bunch of information, which is continuously being updated.

By clearing information, I make way for divine inspiration. It is a great act of healing to be constantly aware and clear away unwanted information that affects my physical body, mental well-being, and emotional health. I can do this using the words "release" and "allow" in the following way, e.g. *"I* **release** *all worry, fear, and self-hatred, and* **allow** *myself to love, appreciate, and accept myself."*

Through releasing old information and perceptions of myself I clear the way for change and transformation at the very deepest level of my being.

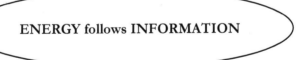

ENERGY follows INFORMATION

Where information goes energy follows. As I transform the information about myself, I genuinely transform my physical body. Through aware and conscious release of information that no longer holds true for me today, I can become whoever I choose to be tomorrow.

Angel Belief

AS I CHANGE THE INFORMATION ABOUT MYSELF, I CHANGE AND TRANSFORM MY PHYSICAL BODY.

From Elephant to Angel Action

Today begin to be aware of all the information that informs you. Focus on what you believe to be true for you and currently limits you. Use the following intent to free yourself from old information that informs your current physical reality:

"I release . . . (put in whatever you want to release yourself from) *and allow myself to claim* . . . (put in the new qualities you want instead) *to be all that I am."*

For example: *"I release fear, judgment, old views of food, and stagnant energy and allow myself to claim joy, peace, a light free body, and the ability to eat anything I want and to be all that I am."*

DAY 17

Elephant Belief

I AM UNABLE TO LIVE MY FULL POTENTIAL, EXPRESS MY FULL CREATIVITY AND BE UNIQUE.

It's amazing to me, after seeing thousands of clients over more than fifteen years of private practice, I can confidently say that all human problems, physical, mental, and emotional all lead back to unfulfilled potential. Every single health issue that I have worked on in myself and others has led back to each individual not fulfilling and living what they came to Earth to be and do. There is some block stopping them from living the way they really want to live. They fail to create, inspire, and be all they came to be. Instead they create dramas, serve others, and generally believe they have to live a certain way that is not aligned with their inherent passions and personality.

When something blocks my potential (where I am meant to be and what I am meant to be doing) I am living at the level of *problems*.

Therefore, to go back to the realm or level of solutions, I must allow myself to once again align with my human destiny—with that which I came to give and to be in this human existence. And let me make this clear—I choose this in each instance, it is not chosen for me. My destiny is always of my own choosing.

My potential is that which I uniquely have to offer and express in the world and through my life. It is what I am here for—my uniqueness. I personally make a vow today to begin, even if in the smallest of ways, to live the life I was born to live, no more excuses. I will express all that I came to create. When I began writing this book, I resisted fully birthing it. While I was in this state of resistance, I had more illnesses in that year than I have had in my entire life. From almost bursting my appendix to severe back problems, I was a walking mess. As soon as I began writing with gusto, all of my symptoms simply disappeared within a few days. Even food intolerances and severe eczema I was experiencing that year just vanished within a couple of weeks!

I EXPRESS MY FULL POTENTIAL AND CREATIVITY THROUGH LIFE AND ALL OF MY ENDEAVORS. I LIVE MY PASSION EACH AND EVERY DAY.

From Elephant to Angel Action

Write a list of what you love to do for fun—this is your passion list. If you have trouble thinking of things, then think back to what you loved doing when you were between nine and twelve years old. At this age, before puberty hit, you were free to do what you truly liked and loved. Perhaps a clue lies in this time period.

Choose one thing from your passion list to commit to doing at least once a week. This is a wonderful way to incorporate passion and fun back into your life and access your innate creativity. With time, this will begin to infuse all aspects of your life, until eventually all of your life will be lived this way. Your life is then a living creative endeavor.

DAY 18

Elephant Belief

I NEED TO PLAN MY DIET AND EXERCISE REGIME.

The biggest mistake I consistently make with my body and even my life is to plan everything out. General planning is great, but if I plan everything and make myself stick to it, then I am designing my life only with my mind. I have consistently learned that what my mind may think is right for me tomorrow is not always correct. Living a life which is strictly planned and regimented may work for some people, but it certainly does not work for me. I find that I am more likely to break my plan at some point and then feel bad about it. I miss out on the spontaneity that life has to offer and the higher guidance waiting to guide me in every moment. I like to think I am better off when the universe plans for me, because it knows more than I do. The universe always has my bigger interest at heart and its wider perspective ensures my outcomes are far better than I could have ever planned. All I have to do is tap in to see what it plans for me at every moment in time. So, instead of planning, I ask throughout the day: *"What food does my body require RIGHT NOW for ultimate vitality, strength, and overall good health?"* Based on the answer I receive, I then eat what I feel like eating in each and every moment.

A student at one of my workshops asked me one time, *"But if I don't plan, how will I know what I need to buy from the supermarket at the beginning of the week?"* My reply? When I began living from the place of listening to my body, something miraculous occurred—I began to intrinsically KNOW what I would want and need for the week ahead. I just knew what to get from the supermarket. I knew what exercise activity to book in for. I became quite intuitive about what I would want tomorrow, knowing exactly what would serve me best. It is not the same thing however as mental planning. Also, planning is usually based on what someone else thinks I need to do, rather than listening to my internal wisdom. It feels to me as though *knowing* comes from a different part of my brain than where *planning* comes from. Many clients over the years have commented that planning feels as though it comes from the front part of the brain, and inner knowing from either the crown of the head or the back of the head. There's something interesting to contemplate!

I know many people will disagree with this philosophy, and certainly I think planning has its time and place, particularly for people who have never eaten diverse and naturally based food, or have never exercised in their life. These sort of people may need some guidance and planning to set them in the right direction initially.

In regards to exercise and movement, I plan the space, the time, the emptiness where movement and exercise will occur but not necessarily what sort of movement will occur. One time at a boxing exercise class, a fellow participant said to me, *"You are so fit. What is your workout plan? I want to follow it."* The reason why I was so fit was because I only exercised for joy and in order to ensure joy when I exercised. I never planned what I did. In other words there was no plan to tell her about. I just did what felt right for me each day. She looked quite perplexed, as this was probably not a way she had looked at exercise before.

I make a commitment to myself to turn up every day, when I am feeling energetic, to the gym. I love exercising in the morning, as it wakes me up and makes me feel alive for the rest of the day, but I never plan the night before what I will be doing. Sometimes I just walk and read, other times I hit the weights, or do a class, but I always allow myself the dignity and right to choose based on where I am at each and every day, and what my body feels like doing. I respect my body's voice and choice in the matter. Sometimes I even sleep in. Choice is my friend and it sets me free.

In regard to movement, I ask, *"What movement do I need RIGHT NOW to energize my body, activate my metabolism, and make me feel good?"*

I listen to my body. It has a voice—and it is always right!

Most people don't know how to listen!

By planning everything, I lose the vital wisdom available to me in each and every moment. I only need to become a proficient listener. Many people wonder how to hear what it is telling them? When you remove your own prescriptions of what you should be doing, and stop planning, you too will begin to hear.

I hear through my gut, through thinking with the intuitive part of my brain, and through feeling, until eventually I just KNOW and build trust in myself. I believe there are never mistakes, and that I am free to choose again next time. I am always free to choose.

I LISTEN TO MY INNER WISDOM IN EVERY MOMENT AND TRUST THE ANSWERS I RECEIVE.

From Elephant to Angel Action

Pick an area of your life that you always plan out. Spend one whole day without planning it at all. This does not mean you just let this day go haywire. Instead, focus on listening to your inner guidance moment by moment throughout your day. Notice which way worked better for you, the old planning way, or the new spontaneous knowing way.

DAY 19

Elephant Belief

EIGHTY-ONE DAYS IS SUCH A LONG TIME TO UNDERTAKE THIS JOURNEY OF CHANGE. I CAN'T DO IT. IT'S TOO HARD!

Before beginning this journey I looked around to find one woman, just one, who is completely secure, comfortable, and in love with her body. I looked and looked, but even the thinnest women threw away lines like: *"If I could just lose ten pounds, then I'd be the weight I was when I was twenty. Then I'd be happy."* It seems that so many people are living in a constant state of dissatisfaction and rejection of what is true and present in the here and now.

Well, I haven't been able to find such a woman, so today I've decided to BE this woman instead. Today I will continue my eighty-one days of releasing any thoughts, emotions, and beliefs about an imperfect me. Today I will embrace this new way of eating and this new way of being. I will embrace a way of expressing self-love and self-acceptance. I will embrace my best way of being whole and complete, naturally trim, taut, and terrific. It's who I am now I've decided, not some distant far off day. Today is the day.

Will you dare to decide too? Will you take a risk, take a chance, and break free from the crowd? Are you willing to continue on this journey of changing old patterns and beliefs to be free? As you transform your view of yourself, your body will also transform. Let's be deliciously free to eat as we please, trust our bodies, and be healthy and slim. Together let's be that woman I was hunting for, until eventually we become the norm. We set the norm. We are the norm.

Oh, and by the way, some days I think eighty-one days is just too long a time. What about change in twenty-one days, like the now common adage? I know deep down that the influence on me is much too deep and much too strong to be gotten rid of in just twenty-one days. This is a long-term change that involves a long-term commitment to myself. I make this commitment to myself today!

TODAY BEGINS A NEW DAY WITH A NEW APPROACH TO EATING, AND A NEW APPROACH TO ME. I KNOW I CAN DO IT.

From Elephant to Angel Action

Today pay attention to your language about what you wish you had, could be, or could change. When you hear yourself speaking in this way, stop and remember how far you have come in this journey. In order to continue successfully you now need to be impeccable with your word, and speak only the good and positive about yourself. Begin today to be a person that is at peace with yourself, self-loving and secure. Be happy today and you will attract more happiness into your life. You attract more of what you are, not what you want.

Get naked and look at your whole body in the mirror today and say to your body, *"I love you today just the way you are."* Change born in self-love and acceptance is the only real and lasting change.

DAY 20

Elephant Belief

I EAT WHAT MY MIND WANTS TO EAT, RATHER THAN WHAT MY BODY WANTS TO EAT. I EAT WHAT THE WEIGHT LOSS EXPERTS SAY I SHOULD EAT, AND I STILL DON'T LOSE WEIGHT.

Sometimes it is difficult to know whether I am really choosing food that my body wants to eat, or whether I am eating with my mind. While it does not matter which, the limitation of choosing just with my mind is that I am so conditioned with what it has been told is good or bad food, and what I should and shouldn't eat. The advice of the experts however is often a passing trend. One day I am told low fat is the way to lose weight, then it's the fault of carbohydrates and I need to add rather than eliminate fat. Soon, I often joke, the experts will be telling me that lettuce is really fattening too! Where does it end, and who am I to believe in a world now saturated with experts?

I, too, could be called an expert, but instead of being an expert, I think of myself more as a guide helping others to become their own experts. I am the only expert for me, and so is each person for himself. We are all expert number one for ourselves. All the other people in my life are what I call information providers. They provide me with information. It is my job to discern what information serves me and what does not. All information is measured against the inherent internal wisdom within myself.

In order to begin eating from within again, I will begin to catch myself when I am choosing food based on what the world thinks is most slimming at the time. I watch for when I begin using words like "should," "have to," "good," and "bad." These words are indicating to me, I am choosing with my conditioned thinking. Instead I set myself free to eat whatever I choose to eat, and I pay attention to how my body feels after I have eaten the food. How my body responds to certain foods is the best possible guide. It will inform me whether my food choice has energized me or made me feel tired. Then I will know what works best for individual me, each and every time.

I LISTEN TO WHAT MY BODY WANTS TO EAT EACH AND EVERY MOMENT, AND SEE HOW I FEEL AFTER EATING AS MY GUIDE TO FUTURE EATING.

From Elephant to Angel Action

Today pay attention to how you feel after each thing you eat. Just for today keep a journal of what you ate, when you ate it, and how you felt after eating it. Write in your journal why you picked that particular food to eat. This will begin to show you when you eat from an external expert perspective versus from your own internal wisdom. When did you feel best? Did you feel better eating what you wanted to eat or when you ate what you thought you should eat?

Remember your body can react to foods differently on different days. It may depend on the season, quality of food, and your health. This is another reason you need to discern how your body is responding to varying foods in each moment.

DAY 21

REST DAY

Today I praise my hips, pelvis, lower back, and the entire lower region of my body. I give thanks for all that it does for me and acknowledge its beauty and strength. I release all that these parts of my body hold and no longer need. Extra stubborn weight on the hips represents a lack of balance in serving others versus serving myself. I heal this in me today using the A.N.G.E.L principle.

I remember to have gratitude and to show this appreciation for all the people in my life who love and help me. I acknowledge both my masculine and feminine qualities and affirm to myself that they are both equally important to me. I am my own best support and speak positive things about myself.

Days of rest are days where much is happening below the perception of the five senses. They are days where I change on a cellular level and allow my true self to come forward a little more each time. Days of rest are dynamic days and as I recognize this I continue to build them into my life on a regular basis.

DAY 22

Elephant Belief

I NEED TO FOLLOW THE RULES OF THE DAY IN ORDER TO FIT IN.

It's not about the food. I realize now it never was. The food is just my vessel, my way of reaching for the things I really want in life. Nor is it about my body. The truth is the only reason it matters to me if I'm thin, attractive, fit, and healthy is because I believe I need these things to give me something, and to make me feel special. Whatever this something is, it is all about feeling good about myself, appreciating and ultimately loving myself. Why do I, therefore, feel so pressured to look a certain way? Why do I have to look a certain way that society dreamed up? In the 1500s and 1600s a plump body was considered beautiful as it was a sign of wealth and stature and there are still communities around the world today where overweight men and women are prized. In these times or places, I bet they beat themselves up psychologically for not eating enough and were mad at their bodies for not gaining weight fast enough!

At the end of the day I want to fit in to the rules of the day and, when I can't, I rebel. That's why much of society is made up of conformists that watch what they eat, weigh themselves regularly, are slim enough and would instantly make themselves thinner if they were given a magic wand! I was amazed recently when speaking to several people at the gym about exercising and they all said they hate working out so hard, but they do it, because it is what they believe they need to do in order to look good. This is how men and women that love and care about themselves are meant to be, isn't it?

On the other hand, the rebels are often those people who tried to follow the group norm, but failed every time and just gave up trying. They assume something is wrong with them, so they eventually rebel against the rules of society, eat whatever they want, judge themselves for it, and then punish themselves some more by eating lots of extra food unnecessarily. Occasionally trying to salvage themselves, they try some new theory or diet and eventually end up back in the rebel patch.

Both types think if they were set free in life with no food rules, body rules, or health rules, they would drop dead from too much chocolate or never exercise again.

Is there something wrong with the motivator here? What happened to coming back to trust in ourselves and doing what is fun and joyful? I find returning to the place of love, pleasure, and enjoyment in life will always create a natural balance in myself, my body, and my life.

Angel Belief

I RELEASE THE NEED TO FOLLOW EXTERNAL RULES SET BY SOCIETY AND INSTEAD CREATE MY OWN RULES BASED ON MY OWN INTERNAL WORLD.

From Elephant to Angel Action

Instead of using your usual rules to motivate yourself today, aim to be guided by pleasure. The aim today is to help you understand that being guided by what feels pleasurable does not mean losing all that you have or giving up on yourself. Pleasure only leads to more joy and joy leads to more true and lasting success. You don't necessarily need to exercise at a painful threshold, eat food that is boring, or even stay at a job that you hate because it is required to fit into society.

Imagine moving in pleasurable ways, eating in pleasurable ways, and doing something you love and getting paid for it? This is possible. Today is the beginning of a new way of looking at your current choices and creating some healthier new rules for yourself.

DAY 23

Elephant Belief

COMPARED TO OTHER PEOPLE, I AM FAT.

I wonder how many people do not use gyms or public places to exercise because they feel very self-conscious about the current state of their body? At places like gyms, where everyone is so concerned about how they look, I can often feel like everyone is comparing me to the perfect body and sizing me up. This doesn't just happen at the gym however. Whenever I go out in public, I notice some people are fatter and some are thinner than me, and that others are noticing me in the same way. I might feel really good about myself as I watch the many obese people on *The Biggest Loser* television show, and then feel really overweight as I watch the Miss Universe competition.

I remind myself that I am not in a universal competition for who can have the better body or the skinnier body. I am not in a secret competition where I win a prize, and I need not travel my whole life comparing myself to others. I received an e-mail one time, that was being circulated, which showed photos of extremely obese people. The friend that sent it wrote, *"Watch this to feel good about yourself! We're not so fat after all."*

Amused, I pondered whether I really wanted to compare myself to suffering obese people in order to feel good about my own body? Can't I just feel good about myself, just because, for no particular reason and not at the expense of someone else? Judging myself against others may seem like a great way to feel good about myself in the short term, but at the end of the day it serves no constructive purpose. We all have our own unique body, face, likes, and dislikes. To compare myself is to downgrade the unique and wondrous being that I am. To compare myself to others is literally like comparing apples to oranges. The sooner I give it up, the sooner I can be free to have the best possible body for me. Ignoring what others are doing or what others look like is a wonderful step in claiming the right body for myself.

Angel Belief

MY BODY IS JUST RIGHT FOR ME.
EACH PERSON'S BODY IS JUST RIGHT FOR THEM.
WE ARE ALL BEAUTIFUL AND UNIQUE.

From Elephant to Angel Action

Today go out of your way to compare yourself to other people's bodies. Notice who you think is more attractive than you, skinnier, fatter. Notice what weight you consider to be fat and what weight you think is just right. These are your current perceptions—*not the truth*. As you notice, catch yourself and remind yourself that everyone is *just right*. Decide to be the weight that feels good for you, and has nothing at all to do with how much other people weigh. This is your body, your goal. Say to yourself, *"I am uniquely me. I love myself just as I am."*

DAY 24

Elephant Belief

IT'S SELFISH TO LOOK AFTER MYSELF FIRST.
I NEED TO PUT OTHER PEOPLE FIRST.

If other people could see the human energy field as I see it, they would often see a giant rush of energy leaking from most people. This is because for at least 80 percent of people, or more, their energy pours out to other people. They are giving their energy away, through being attached to the approval of others, wanting to make other people happy, having sympathy for their predicaments, and even healing others. We are taught to do this from childhood. We are taught to make sure that everyone around us is well first, and only then to care for ourselves; otherwise we are being selfish. Too often, however, after we are finished looking after everybody else, there is very little energy left for ourselves.

For years I wondered why so many people that worked in the healing profession seemed to die so young. I was often worried that this would happen to me too, since it seemed every twelve months or so of working intensely with clients, I would get burned out. It wasn't until many years of healing others that I was told by an extraordinary practitioner I consulted, despite the many boundaries I had set up in working with clients, I was giving my energy away to each and every one of them. His view was that I was "addicted to serving humanity." Huh? Isn't this what I was supposed to be doing? After all, much of the self-help and spiritual literature speaks of finding true peace through serving and giving to others. Serving is the highest ideal, right?

At the time, I was completely confused. The practitioner went on to explain that being addicted to helping others is different from sharing my unique talents and gifts with the world. The former puts others first at the cost of myself. The thinking is, *"Giving to others is more important than giving to myself, no matter what the personal cost,"* and it has an addictive quality. I also found it difficult to stop working in the healing profession, no matter how much it disrupted my personal life or my health. I was literally addicted to it. In truth, it fed my self-esteem. My story went something like this: *"What an amazing person I am as I always put other people first and create the most incredible healing in them. I am such an amazingly gifted and special person."* While this is true to some extent, the ego's story is one that required me to prostitute myself for the love and approval of others, which is exactly what I did.

Sharing my unique talents and gifts with the world, on the other hand, is a totally different form of giving. It is giving from a glass totally full, rather than from an empty one. From this place of giving, I know who I am, nurture myself first, and then have so much love overflowing, there is nothing else I could possibly do other than share it with the world.

At some point in my evolution I needed to learn to help others with my actions NOT with my energy. The sign of a "healthy" person, in my experience, is someone who nurtures and loves themselves first, so they have more to give. This sort of person has an energy field that is directed inwards first.

In regards to looking after my body, it is not sufficiently self-nurturing to eat well and exercise regularly. While this is a good beginning, for me it is always the energy that counts first. Where energy goes, all else follows. If my energy is directed inward, then self-nurturing actions follow with loving intent and my body thrives. When I am busy helping everyone else first and my energy is outwardly focused, then exercise and healthy eating may not be enough to bring about a healthy mind, body, and soul.

It brings to mind a client, whom I saw several years ago, who hardly ate a thing all day, exercised regularly, and was quite overweight. She blamed her hormones and metabolism, but for me these things were only presenting limitations to her successful weight loss because of something much deeper. Specifically, she was giving away all of her vital energy to others. While she appeared to be nurturing herself, her intent of self-love was missing. After giving most of her energy away to family and friends, there wasn't much left for herself. After only a couple of sessions she was a different person. Armed with her new understanding and a new commitment to herself first and foremost, she not only went on to lose over sixty pounds, but she was more present than ever for her loved ones. When I nurture myself first, there is so much more of me to give. I benefit and everyone else benefits too.

Angel Belief

I PUT MYSELF FIRST, MAKING SURE I AM FULL OF LOVE AND ENERGY. I NURTURE MYSELF AS A PRIORITY. WHEN I AM FULL I HAVE MORE TO GIVE TO OTHERS.

From Elephant to Angel Action

Susan Tate in her book *Wellness Wisdom: 31 Ways to Nourish Your Mind, Body and Spirit* suggests creating a wellness bucket. I just love this idea, so today I am going to borrow Susan's idea and inspire you to do the same. She suggests drawing a bucket on a large piece of paper and writing or drawing inside it all of the things that fill your wellness bucket, such as meditation, spending time with friends, and so on. On the outside of the bucket, write all the things and people that poke holes in your bucket. Susan refers to these, as the things that make your bucket leak.

I would like you to also expand on this approach by writing a list of actions that you can take from today onward to minimize or totally delete some or all of the stressors found outside of your bucket. The less of these there are, the less your energy leaks to outside sources and to other people.

DAY 25

Elephant Belief

I NEED OTHER PEOPLE TO SUPPORT ME IN ORDER TO LOSE WEIGHT SUCCESSFULLY.

Weight loss is a quiet inner job, not a desperate outer one. What this means is, I will be more successful at losing weight when I do it privately for me, and do not need to tell the world. I do not need to convince anyone other than myself. I do not require anyone else's support, other than my own. I need only do it quietly as I go about living with humbleness and grace. Even eating in this new way as espoused by this book is something that I need not share with others straight away. I am doing it for me, so I do it quietly, believing in myself along the way and allowing other people to do what they think is best for them. While we can gain momentum in groups, they can also sabotage our momentum. Losing weight with the revolutionary new approach in this book will not be everyone's cup of tea. Many people will not agree it is possible, as they will not as yet have made the quantum leap in thinking that you and I are making.

While I am learning all of these new ways of being, I am aware that I am more vulnerable and the new beliefs I am adopting are also still vulnerable. These new beliefs are not yet planted into the ground, and not yet strong enough. Someone else planting the seed of doubt at this very fragile time for me could destroy all of my progress and cause me to doubt myself and this whole new way of relating to food. Therefore, I allow my new weight-loss journey to be private, quiet, peaceful, and serene. When I begin receiving all the compliments about how good I'm looking and how comfortable and relaxed in my eating I am, then I can choose to share with others my new eating approach, if it feels right for me to do so.

Making changes to my mind and body in this internal manner brings better results. I don't need anyone else's approval. The only sacred contract is between me, myself, and I.

I remember the first time I decided to partake in a special Chinese method of fasting. This involved having no food or water for as many days as I could manage. This method required me to imagine drinking and eating as often as I liked throughout the day, but no real food or water was permitted. On this first undertaking, I went around telling everyone I was doing this. Now, most people thought I was mad, while others I told were clearly envious. Needless to say by the end of the second day, I had given up. The energies and thoughts of other people were confusing me. I started to doubt that this was a beneficial practice at all. Following this first attempt, a few weeks later I went on to fast again using this same method and this time did so for six whole days without any food or water. It was easy, I could have easily kept going, and I felt better than ever. During those six days very few and select people knew I was fasting. I kept going to the gym, kept doing all of my normal activities, and no one suspected a thing. I kept my power to myself, rather than allowing other people to interfere with my power. This is self-empowerment!

Angel Belief

> ## I CAN LOSE WEIGHT ON MY OWN.
> ## I NEED NOT SHARE IT WITH OTHERS.
> ## I KEEP MY POWER TO MYSELF AND AM
> ## EMPOWERED IN THE PROCESS.

From Elephant to Angel Action

Set an intention today to limit who you tell about undertaking this new approach other than your very closest confidantes, if even them. Remind yourself you do not need to convince yourself that this works by convincing others that it does. You just need to do it for yourself. Commit to supporting yourself and know that this is enough for you to be successful.

DAY 26

Elephant Belief

I CAN'T BE TRUSTED AROUND "BAD" FOOD.

I was visiting with a friend today who described to me how little she eats in a day. She shared this quite proudly, and when I suggested that this might not be so good for her body, she went on to say that she loves eating this way and this is what she genuinely wants to keep doing.

Of course, I do try most of the time not to look deeply into my friends' issues with my medical intuitive abilities as I might with a client, but on this occasion I really could not help but see in her energy field that she was very much lying to me and to herself. Her energy clearly showed me that she loved to eat a lot, was scared of food and its effects, and that being thin was of utmost importance to her self-esteem. She needed to be thin, even if the cost was her health.

When I probed her a little more, she continued to attest to the fact that even if she could eat anything in the world, she would still eat as she currently did. Later on during our visit she asked the children whether they wanted a packet of chocolate cookies to eat. They answered *no* to which she replied, *"Good, because if I'd opened them, then I would have eaten the whole packet."* This didn't sound at all congruent with her original story!

The point I am making is, I want to always be honest with myself, rather than pretending I don't like the occasional bad food. If chocolate chip cookies are what I really love and want right this minute, then I will allow myself to eat them, thus avoiding the binge eating that results from deprivation. I can be trusted around bad food because there is no food that is actually bad, and I trust myself to eat it.

Sometimes I want what I want because I think I cannot have it. Like my friend with the chocolate cookies, who pretended she only loved eating healthy food; secretly she was longing for those chocolate cookies. Why else would she not trust herself around them? Was she frightened that she may sit around all day and eat chocolate cookies? Chocolate cookies for my friend represent more than food. They represent the real longings of her heart that she feels she cannot have. She does not trust herself to live life the way she really wants to, in case this means she stops being the responsible mother and wife that is expected of her.

When I break free from my fear of food I am also breaking free from my fear of life. To not trust myself around food, in fear that if I start eating I may never stop, shows a much deeper longing of my heart. I am not giving myself what I really want in life.

Furthermore the whole chocolate-cookie scenario also reveals a much deeper belief of *"I don't deserve to eat the whole packet of chocolate cookies because I will be punished for it later with weight gain."* Life translation of this is *"I do not deserve to have what I want in life because there is pain involved at some point."* What a limiting belief to engage in. Time to let it go!

Angel Belief

I CAN EAT ANYTHING I WANT AND AS MUCH AS I WANT, AND I TRUST MYSELF AROUND ALL FOOD.

From Elephant to Angel Action

On a fresh piece of paper, make two columns. In column one, list any foods that you know right now you like and on the other side write all the foods you can think of that you do not like. As the day progresses, pay attention to what foods you genuinely like or dislike. Being honest today is the beginning of being honest with yourself about everything in your life.

Now make another list with two columns: one listing aspects of your life that you love and one listing aspects of your life that you hate. What would you change if you could? Honesty is the first step toward change and transformation.

DAY 27

Elephant Belief

I CAN'T LOSE WEIGHT BECAUSE THERE ARE TOO MANY TOXINS IN MY BODY, I AM LACKING CERTAIN VITAMINS AND MINERALS, OR THERE IS SOMETHING WRONG WITH MY HORMONES.

In my view of health, after more than ten years of treating people with almost every possible health condition, I have found that nothing happens to the body by accident. There is always an underlying reason for all that unfolds in the human body, and that reason begins at the level of belief, crosses through thoughts and emotions, and eventually lands in the physical realm. In my view of the body, any excess toxins, hormonal issues, and deficiencies in vitamins and minerals still stem back to a weakness at the level of thought, feeling, or emotion. I am yet to meet an overweight person, or an ill person, who is happy, joyous, forgiving, has a near perfect outlook on life, a high self-esteem, and loves every part of their life. Generally, I can always find a crack in any exterior.

What follows is a very brief list of some of the most important and often lacking vitamins and minerals, as well as toxins and their relationship to special mind centers of the body. These twelve mind centers are located in various locations on the body and are fully explained in the book *The Healing Secrets of the Ages* by Catherine Ponder.

The relationship I have drawn below is based on my own research, and while there is no scientific evidence to prove that my correlations are correct, it has proven correct for me over many years in clinical practice. I use this only as a guide as it is a fairly generalized list. Whenever there is an imbalance in my body I use this list to see whether there is something in my thinking that also needs recalibrating.

Faith	Do I have faith in myself, my purpose, and life in general? Do I have faith in a higher power?
	Lack of faith can result in either too much or too little estrogen.
	Solution: I imagine the color blue bathing the center of my brain where the pineal gland is found. I feel this blue infusing this part of my brain with purpose and faith. I allow the blue to bring my faith back both for myself as well as for a higher power—my deepest inner power.
Strength	Do I really know who I am and do I have the strength to be myself no matter what? Have I the inner strength to do what I want to do rather than what others expect of me?
	Lack of strength can lead to a deficiency of either vitamin E, B1, and/or carnitine.
	Solution: I imagine the color red bathing the strength center in my body, in the small of my back, in the middle of the adrenal glands. I feel this red bringing confidence and strength back into my body and back into my life.
Judgment	Have I been judging myself or others harshly lately? Is this judgment holding me back and condemning me rather than motivating me forward?
	Judgment can lead to a deficiency in magnesium. It can also lead to antimony toxicity.
	Solution: I imagine the color gold infusing the stomach and solar plexus areas of my body, clearing and energizing my pancreas, clearing away all judgment of myself and others.

Love	Do I feel and express unconditional love for myself and others or am I limited by bitterness, resentment, and unhappiness? Do I hold on to the past or forgive and forget?
	Lack of unconditional love for myself and lack of forgiveness for others can lead to a deficiency of vitamin D and/or vitamin A.
	Solution: I imagine the color green in my heart area. I feel this color clearing away all grief, sadness, resentment, and barriers to joy in this area, and infusing my thymus gland with positivity and passion.
Power	Do I use my words to reflect the positive and the good about myself and others or am I speaking words of negativity and condemnation? Do I always speak the truth?
	Lack of power can lead to a deficiency of zinc and/or iron. It can also be linked with excess cadmium.
	Solution: I imagine the color orange bathing my throat and thyroid gland, giving me the gift of truth. I speak my truth and share words of love about myself and others.
Imagination	Am I deliberately directing my imagination to create what I desire? Do I dedicate time each day to hearing, knowing, seeing, and feeling the messages of the Divine, which is imagining for me?
	A lack of utilizing your imagination can lead to a deficiency in molybdenum.
	Solution: I imagine the color yellow in between my eyes, correcting my pituitary gland, and activating my imagination. I allow this color to bring life back into my body and into my life.

Understanding	Do I feel connected to a higher power within myself? Do I listen and act upon my intuition and follow the guidance and wisdom of my inner knowing?

A lack of understanding can lead to a deficiency in manganese.

Solution: I imagine the color violet pouring into my forehead and into the front of my brain, connecting me with my inner intuitive ability. I allow this purple to fill my entire head and body. I am back online to hearing and knowing my own inner guidance and wisdom.

Will	Does my will follow my intuitive guidance, bringing action to my guidance, or does it fight and argue through logic? Do I live through willpower alone without a clear idea of my correct individual path?

Living through willpower alone can lead to a deficiency of B12. It can also be linked to excess copper.

Solution: I imagine in the front of my brain the color indigo infusing itself through my head. I allow this color to release the need for the will center to always be in charge. I allow the color indigo to heal this part of my brain, bringing peace and harmony back into my body.

Order	Are my thoughts and feelings orderly or disorderly? Are my environment and my relationships ordered and peaceful or is there always drama and disorder in my life and surroundings?

Lack of order can lead to a deficiency in selenium.

Solution: I imagine the color navy blue bathing my abdominal area, right behind my navel, bringing order back into my body and into my entire life.

| Zeal | Do I have the enthusiasm and freedom to express all of my ideas and talents? Am I resisting or fighting something in my life or is joy consistently what I live for? Am I resistant to new ideas, new ways of doing things, and a new way of being in my body and in the world, based on pleasure and joy? |

Lack of zeal can lead to a lack of progesterone.

Solution: I imagine the color pink infusing the back of my neck at the base of the brain, bringing joy, enthusiasm, and vigor into my body, mind, and soul. I allow this color to keep pouring into me until my neck feels relaxed and renewed.

Elimination Do I hold on to people, things, and attitudes that are no longer necessary for my highest good? Do I have trouble surrendering my life to the divine self that is ready to give me all that I want and more? Is control a central part of my psyche?

Lack of elimination can lead to a deficiency in vitamin C and/ or vitamin B6.

Solution: I imagine the color brown bathing the elimination organs in my body, allowing me to release all the things I have been holding on to. It is time to let go. I allow this color to keep spreading through this part of my body until I find myself taking a deep breath.

Life Am I feeling tired and fatigued or lacking in energy? Am I living my purpose and life mission each and every day? Am I living my life or am I too busy serving others at the expense of myself or merely for money?

Lack of life power can lead to a deficiency in coenzyme Q10.

Solution: I imagine the color white in my reproductive organs bringing back full energy, creativity, and a sense of purpose into my life. I allow this color to spread throughout my entire body until it fills me and spreads out of my body filling the entire room with white light. I say yes to the purpose that is currently nagging at my soul.

Angel Belief

THERE IS AN EMOTIONAL SOLUTION TO EVERY PHYSICAL PROBLEM.

From Elephant to Angel Action

Tune in intuitively, or even guess, which of the above power centres are causing issues for you right now. Use the appropriate solution offered and allow yourself to bath in the color suggested until you feel yourself taking a deep breath. As soon as this deep breath naturally occurs, then the exercise is complete. If you have time, you can do all twelve just to be sure. This exercise is also included as a meditation on my CD "You Can Channel Too!"

Angel Belief

THERE IS AN EMOTIONAL SOLUTION TO EVERY PHYSICAL PROBLEM.

From Elephant to Angel Action

Tune in intuitively, or even guess which of the power centers are causing issues for you right now. Use the appropriate solution offered and allow yourself to bathe in the color suggested until you feel yourself taking a deep breath. As soon as this deep breath naturally occurs, then the exercise is complete. If you have time, you can do all twelve just to be sure.

DAY 28

REST DAY

Today is a day of rest. I acknowledge and praise myself for how far I have come on this journey of inner and outer transformation. I am amazing, powerful, and strong. I give gratitude to myself for being brave enough to look my beliefs straight in the face and challenge them. I am genuinely committed to myself and now is the time to more fully commit to this process no matter how long it takes for me. I know I will get there when I am supposed to.

DAY 29

Elephant Belief

I AM UNABLE TO STOP EATING SO MUCH PROCESSED FOOD.

In my experience working with clients who want to lose weight, I have noticed that they tend to focus on what needs to be avoided or eliminated. My personal philosophy is that nothing needs to be eliminated at all because all food is good food, and all food is neutral. Instead I shift my focus from what not to eat to the foods I would like to add more of into my diet. I never try to eliminate any food I find myself wanting to reduce, as I inevitably end up wanting to eat it even more than before. If for example I find at times I do not like the way I am physically feeling after eating chocolate, but love eating it and cannot seem to give it up, I focus instead on eating more fruit. Then I find I no longer actually want the chocolate anymore. I use the **Add Instead of Delete Principle**. When I focus on adding nutrients to my everyday eating, my body naturally begins to feel good and all false cravings easily disappear on their own, rather than through mental force.

Below are a few of the powerhouse foods that I love to add to my everyday eating for added nutrition. I can still eat anything I want and feel great. Adding these foods however lets my body know that I am feeding it all the nutrition that it needs rather than only feeding my mind's needs. I remind myself often that the key is to add foods rather than forcing myself to delete foods. Things that I no longer need will fall away by themselves. I also find that as my nutritional needs are met, my body stops being so hungry all the time. Constant hunger can mean that my body is hungry for vitamins and minerals.

My nutritional cupboard includes:

Nuts and seeds

Packed with nutrients such as B vitamins, fiber, antioxidants, and more. A great way to increase their vitamin levels even more is to soak them in water overnight and then rinse them well. They can be stored in the refrigerator for up to a week.

Flaxseed oil

A great source of omega-3 fatty acids.

Hemp oil

Has the ideal ratio of omega-6 and omega-3 fatty acids.

Young coconuts, coconut oil, and coconut flour

Contains medium chain triglycerides, which are converted by the liver to energy.

Chlorella

Is 65 percent protein and has a high amount of essential fatty acids, vitamins, minerals, enzymes and nineteen amino acids. Chlorella is wonderful for detoxing, too.

Maca powder

This is one of my favorites! A root vegetable from Peru, Maca helps the adrenal glands to heal from stress, helps to construct serotonin, and can assist in balancing the hormonal system. I have this four days a week and it has transformed my health and my exercise recovery rate. It's best not to take every day as it loses its efficacy.

Pseudo-grains like amaranth, buckwheat, wild rice, and quinoa

These grains and flours are packed with nutrients and are gluten free. I love to use them in my baking and know I am eating so many nutrients (there are just too many to list). I make cakes out of a combination of them, and so when I'm eating my cake I'm also getting a nutritional hit!

Sea vegetables such as dulse, nori, and kelp

They are packed with minerals which are hard to find in other foods, and electrolytes that help to keep us hydrated for longer.

Fermented foods

The addition of fermented foods to my diet has done extraordinary things for my digestion. Fermented foods include miso, fermented drinks (that I buy ready made), cultured vegetables, yogurt, and kefir. Fermented foods are rich in good bacteria and, added to your diet, will give you natural acidophilus and aid the body to eliminate toxins and heal itself. I particularly eat them in Autumn to help my digestion.

Chia seeds

These super seeds have eight times more omega-3 EFAs than salmon, packed with eighteen amino acids, are a complete protein, having five times more iron than spinach, and are packed with calcium and magnesium.

There are many other wonderful nutrient dense superfoods to be sure, but I have just briefly mentioned some of my absolute favorites. The point is to add more nutritional foods to your diet and observe how your food choices change naturally.

Angel Belief

AS I ADD MORE NUTRITIOUS FOODS TO MY EVERY DAY EATING, FOODS I NO LONGER NEED FALL AWAY ON THEIR OWN.

From Elephant to Angel Action

Today I dare you to seek out just one of the foods I have listed above and try incorporating it into your diet for a week. Notice what effect it has on you after eating it. Notice how you feel after incorporating it into your eating for a week. Has anything changed naturally in your cravings and food choices? Make a list of five more foods you can add into your eating plan to add vitamins and minerals and vitality to your diet. Maybe add an extra protein source, extra vegetables, or nuts. Allow these five choices to come from within you, rather than from what the experts claim you need to add.

DAY 30

Elephant Belief

I FEEL VERY UNGROUNDED AT TIMES AND NOT VERY PRESENT IN MY BODY.

How many people, I wonder, walk around in their head or even in the clouds instead of being fully grounded and present in the body? To be grounded means to be in the body fully and to feel the aliveness of it. When I am grounded I feel very connected to what I physically feel and more aware of what my body is saying in every moment. I am fully present with it and in it. Many people I meet, however, are not.

Today while meditating I discovered there are times, due to being unable to cope with emotional overwhelm, when I step out of my body and sort of leave it behind. Where do I go? Well, somewhere other than here and now. Perhaps I am in the past or in the future, but it feels like a lofty sort of place. During this meditation I discovered that my body during such times feels unloved and abandoned.

I used this meditation opportunity to apologize to my body. I made a vow to it that I would forge a close partnership with it. Like a marriage vow, I promised to love, respect, and listen to it and know it is capable of the extraordinary! I also began to spend a few minutes throughout the day focusing on my breathing. Through doing this I am not trying to make my breathing any deeper, but rather just paying attention to it. I also spent a few moments throughout the day concentrating on the aliveness of my body. In feeling the aliveness, I just took a few minutes to feel the energy of my feet, my legs, and so on. Doing these simple acts helped me ground back consciously into my body.

There are many energy techniques, such as visualizing a red cord from the base of the spine going into Earth, that many use to ground themselves, but I believe that in order for grounding to be whole and complete, I need a more organic approach. Through the breath-and-body-awareness exercise done for only a few minutes here and there I am training my body to be grounded always.

At one of my workshops, there was a participant who said she didn't want to be in her body. She liked being ungrounded because heaven felt safer and it was where she wanted to feel she was. I asked her why she was even here on Earth in this case, to which she replied that she didn't want to be here at all and wanted to commit suicide to be back in heaven.

It was then that I found the following words surprisingly coming out of my mouth, *"Go then. Go back home, but where exactly are you going to go? There is no place out 'there' that is better than here! There is no heaven, outside of you, that is more than the Divine that lives in this moment. You do not realize yet that you brought heaven with you. Heaven is here and now, in your body and in your life. You are searching for it 'up there,' but the only place it is found is here and now. You brought it all with you."* These words shocked us both, and as they did, I saw the part of her that was always trying to escape to some better reality come back fully into her body. She became fully grounded and went on to live a much happier present life.

When I escape my body to avoid what is here and now, I abandon myself. It can only be through this moment and being fully present and alive in it that I can fully transform.

Angel Belief

I ALLOW MYSELF TO BE FULLY PRESENT IN MY BODY AND GROUNDED AT ALL TIMES.

From Elephant to Angel Action

Begin this practice today by paying attention to your breathing. Just stop what you are doing and observe it. Then pay attention to actually feeling your body. Begin feeling the aliveness and the energy in your feet, in you legs, moving up through your hips, torso, hands, arms, shoulders, and head. Feel yourself as one whole living being. Then imagine this feeling spreading out even beyond your physical body to include the pulsing of your energy body. This is you. This is all of you, here and now.

DAY 31

Elephant Belief

I AM MY BODY.

How easy it is to forget who I really am! After all, it is so difficult to define. It just is. It is big and wild and free. It is unfettered and has no boundaries. It is me. It is my soul, my spirit, my light. Instead of accepting this, I am tempted by the world to give myself all of the labels I have worked so hard to attain. I am tempted to call myself a mother, an author, a healer, and so many other things. When I momentarily forget and take these labels to be who I am, I also take what I see to be who I am, namely my body and all that it represents. I become that person in the mirror and all the many labels attached to her. I become all of the labels attached to me.

I know what it is to be ugly. Growing up, something unusual happened to my jaw, as the right side kept growing. As the familiar young face I had always liked began to disappear, and the face that was so often teased at school for being a "jabber jaw" appeared, I began to think that girl in the mirror was ugly. I became the label. I thought and believed it was who and what I was.

Some years later I undertook a harrowing six hours of surgery to correct my face, and in the process lost a great amount of weight due to being unable to eat. Recovering from this surgery just as I was beginning my college studies, I found myself suddenly not only with a pretty face but a thin body to match. I began receiving complimentary looks from men, and as I felt a new power I had never known in school, I suddenly became the body and face I now carried. I believed I was my body, and my looks, hence it was important to keep them at any cost. In a world gone mad with the power of the outer appearance, I experienced first hand what going from ugly to attractive created in both how I was treated and how I treated and thought of myself.

I'm sure the wounds of this life experience still sit with me somewhere in my psyche, influencing my food choices, my relationship with others, and my relationship with my self. I am an avid reader, and have read many spiritual texts all espousing the view that I am not my body, but pure spirit in this wonderful vehicle for a short period of time. I understand this mentally, yet somewhere inside of me I must believe it still counts to be externally attractive and certainly slim. It is important to me that I am, especially if I want to be loved in the world.

In this deeper understanding today, I release this need in me, knowing that when I no longer think I am my body, and need or absolutely require myself to be thin, that I will just be thin anyway. Whatever thin means for me, I will allow it to be what it is without the need to always have what I consider perfection. I am not my body! I am so much more, and I acknowledge this real part of me today and allow all else to fall away. I will look after my vehicle but it is not what or who I am. I honor it and release it to a higher power. I am free to be me at any weight. I am always me and I am more than my body.

Angel Belief

I AM MORE THAN MY BODY.
I AM LIGHT, LOVE, AND SPIRIT
FIRST AND FOREMOST.

From Elephant to Angel Action

Pay attention today to all of the roles that you ascribe to. Remember this is not who you really are. Allow yourself to acknowledge these many roles and every time you catch yourself taking your roles too seriously say to yourself, *"This is not who I really am. Who I am is indefinable."* As you begin to realize that most of your life is spent playing pretend roles, you will free yourself from them.

Write a list of why it is so important to you to be thin. Why is being thin seen as more valuable to you, more important sometimes than the deeper essence of who you really are? Next to each reason write *"Pure spirit is all that I really am. Nothing else is real."* Write it over and over again next to each of your reasons. Now you will remember.

DAY 32

Elephant Belief

I AM ATTACHED TO CERTAIN THINGS AND CANNOT LET GO.

One of the interesting things I've noticed is that whatever I am attached to entraps me and I find myself eventually imprisoned by it.

At one point, when I was forever afflicted with health issues, many friends and practitioners I consulted recommended that I give up my martial arts training and gym exercise until I got better. However, I just could not give them up. I am sure at the time I knew deep down it would help me to get better, but the image of a strong, sexy, lethal me was too good to risk losing. I had to hold on to it at any cost. I kept moving toward it to the detriment of my intuitive voice. I was completely attached to both, and could not accept stopping as a possibility. I could not, and would not, let go. Fighting to hold on, I heard once again from a revered Chinese practitioner not to push myself in exercise too much. Finally I had to admit I was attached, addicted to the so-called benefits I attributed to these practices.

Whenever I am attached to anything in life, it entraps me, and so long as this is the case, I am not fluid enough to know what I really need to be doing. When I let go, I know on a deeper level what I really want and what is truly best for me. When I make space for something new to come into my life, I find my life flows again with balance and serenity. When I am struggling to make something happen that I think I need, my attachment often clouds my judgment. Besides, when I let go and give something up, if it truly is meant for me, it will simply come back again.

I ponder today the many other things I am attached to in regards to food, but also in the wider scope of my life. I consider what people, places, jobs, habits, and routines I would struggle to let go of. I know I need to give myself permission to let them go. Having no attachments does not mean I am cold hearted and shallow. Instead it means that I value these things immensely while at the same time acknowledging nothing is permanent in life. They all will pass as I will one day pass from this world also. Understanding and making peace with this fact allows me to live more freely and joyously today, being attached to nothing, but having extreme gratitude for everything!

Angel Belief

I AM ATTACHED TO NOTHING.
MY HAPPINESS RELIES ON NOTHING EXTERNAL.
IT IS A CHOICE THAT I MAKE.

From Elephant to Angel Action

Close your eyes and ask that you be shown all of the things you are attached to with cords connecting these things physically to some part of your body. Imagine these cords are real and are connected to your actual body. Note where they are located on your body. Imagine using a sword of white light to sever these cords. Imagine them being cut away as easily as a hot knife through butter. As they melt away, imagine white light melting away any remnants of the cords still attached to your body. Imagine them melting away, no matter how deep inside you they run. Fill the empty space left behind with a beautiful emerald green light. This light is the color of love and healing. You are free from all attachments. Feel golden light covering you and reenergizing you.

DAY 33

Elephant Belief

I "SHOULD," "MUST," "HAVE TO" DO CERTAIN THINGS AND BE A CERTAIN WAY.

Whenever I hear myself utter the words "have to," "must," or "should," this is a signal that there is a limiting belief hindering my personal growth. There is nothing that I should, have to, or must do. I am always free to choose. When I use these words it is a sign to me that I am living from a deep rule given to me, rather than signaling a choice I am making. When I catch myself saying these words (and I do several times a day), I replace the words with "I choose to." This lets me off the hook and then I can do these things five times better and faster. If on the other hand I don't really choose to at all, then I don't do it.

I wonder how many people I hear in a day saying, *"I should eat more fruits and vegetables."* Whenever my husband or children use one of these words, I always reply with, *"According to who?"* Whose is the voice of the should, have to, and must? It's rarely my voice. It's the voice of the person I have made the external expert in my head, but it's not my voice at all. Anytime I do a "should" when I don't really want to it costs me vital energy. An accumulation of such actions creates a profoundly negative deficit on my health.

Using these words also shows me that I am setting myself up to fail. Even though I might say "should" all day long, I rarely carry out the "should," and then feel like a failure. So instead I will choose with faith and conviction in myself, and march along knowing I am free. When I make such a choice free from the restrictions of having to, then I know I make a genuine choice for me.

Angel Belief

I AM FREE TO CHOOSE WHAT I DO AND HOW I DO EVERYTHING IN MY LIFE.

From Elephant to Angel Action

Catch yourself today saying the words "must," "have to," or "should." Do you really "have to" do anything? Decide if you really want to do these things, and if you do decide you "choose to," then do so from a place of full empowerment. If you do not really want to do these things, then let them go and move along. Notice how many times you use these limiting words, and how you feel in your body when you do. Make a new choice today. Train your mind to say to yourself, *"According to who?"* when you find yourself trying to convince yourself you really should!

DAY 34

Elephant Belief

I FIND IT DIFFICULT TO MAKE DECISIONS AND TO KNOW WHAT I REALLY WANT.

There was a period of about a year where I spent most of the year in complete confusion, questioning everything in my life. I was confused as to what I really wanted. So many possibilities and I didn't feel sure what made me happy anymore. Such times occur for me usually when change is looming up ahead. Instead of waiting for myself and the universe to match up, I keep trying to decide (this or that?) about everything. One morning as I woke up feeling the usual conflict in my mind and heart, I suddenly had a revelation: the reason I couldn't decide what I really wanted was because I was addicted to the inner turmoil. While it didn't appear that I enjoyed it at the time, something in me fed off this practice. Some part of me feels alive or free while in a constant state of inner confusion. On the other hand maybe I just use it as a way to avoid making life-changing decisions.

While I speak of life decisions here, remember everything I touch upon through these days reflects back into food and my relationship with it. Quite honestly, at the same time as I was going through this inner conflict, my eating habits were just the same. I never knew what I wanted to eat, eating anything and everything because it was there, and never knowing when to stop. I was addicted to the mental drama, the constant internal war going on inside of me.

Eating anything and everything without regard is also a way to avoid making choices in life!

Today when I become aware of myself doing this same thing, I walk away. I decide not to play this mental battle, to no longer participate, and to no longer become trapped in this mental matrix. What this behavior reflects is an internal battle between my intellect and intuition. I know that it is never about the choice, but the drama about the choice. As though this somehow gives me the illusion that, by always having a choice, I am free. I am not. This is not freedom.

When I no longer participate in the drama, I make space for the real answers to arrive. What I have learned the hard way is that I do not receive answers from the universe when I ask questions and then try to force an answer to come. No! Instead, once I ask the question and release it I find my true answers come to me when I am quiet and peaceful inside. Life simply answers my questions with all of the many clues it leaves for me each and every day. I begin to live the answers.

Angel Belief

**KNOWING WHAT I WANT IS EASY AND SIMPLE.
I MAKE DECISIONS WITH EASE AND RELEASE
ALL CONFLICT WITHIN ME.
LIFE ALWAYS SHOWS ME WHAT IS BEST FOR ME.**

From Elephant to Angel Action

When you catch yourself today trying to decide about anything at all, place this matter on a beautiful cloud of light. Allow this light to be like God's altar—a place where all the hard work is done for you. In this place the best possible solution will be brought to you and it will be the perfect outcome, far more perfect than anything you could possibly come up with yourself. Remember to place any dilemma, any internal conflict, any worries, and any decisions required on this white cloud.

Notice how much lighter you feel without having to mentally work these things out for yourself. Notice throughout the week whether more and more clarity comes to you about these issues. Do they somehow resolve themselves? When you release problems in this way, you allow life to bring the answers and solutions you seek. Life loves you and never lets you down.

DAY 35

REST DAY

Today is a day of rest. I feel rejuvenated today. Today I just rest and do things that are frivolous and fun. Today I do nothing at all. I commit to do nothing, and allow myself to just be instead, with faith that all the hard work I have invested in myself so far is paying off and I am transforming in unimaginable ways. Today I simply rest, and praise myself for doing nothing. It can be hard to do nothing as I am so conditioned to always be doing something. Today I purposefully choose to do nothing and enjoy it. The peace and quiet will be well worth it and I will make deeper progress tomorrow and the days that follow will be even more creative and powerful as a result.

DAY 36

I FEEL HOPELESS. WHEN I WAKE UP FEELING NEGATIVE I CANNOT FIND A WAY TO SEE THE LIGHT AGAIN.

I hate feeling emotional. I hate feeling bad, feeling sick, and especially feeling fat. The truth is, I want to feel happy, healthy, energetic, and of course—thin. I feel good when I feel thin. I radiate vibrancy, life, and high self-esteem. It isn't only about boosting my ego. It does indeed help me feel energetic and alive.

Even though today I woke up feeling so low, thinking about it now, I realize it is through the times when I fall that I am led to another bit of life-changing information, another approach I had not thought of before, and another form of inspiration. It is often when I have lost faith in myself and given up that I bother to look for help and actually accept help from others.

Life is about change and adding new things is what keeps me alive. In truth all things, all of my brilliant ways, eventually lose their luster and their efficacy. Newness, learning, and personal growth is and always has been my lifelong endeavor.

So, today, as I have awakened feeling desperate, unhappy, and low, I am going to congratulate myself for this. Thank goodness I'm feeling this way today! How many people say that to themselves when they wake up feeling this way? Feeling this way today is a sign that I am letting go of old ways of thinking and allowing new things, new growth, and new freedom to emerge in me.

The truth is I would never have written this book if I did not once feel low myself. It is only through acceptance and learning through my own difficult times in life that I have grown to now help others. I do not know everything about life, and probably not anyone on Earth does, but as each person learns they can become the beacon for someone else, who has given up, to follow.

Every time I leave the place of love and inner peace, I am destined to return, and each time I return, I return stronger than before, wiser than before, and more alive than ever before.

I KNOW THAT I AM GROWING AND LEARNING EVERY DAY AND WHEN I FEEL HOPELESS I WILL FIND A NEW AND BETTER WAY TO BE IN LOVE AND FAITH ONCE MORE.

From Elephant to Angel Action

Write a letter to yourself for when you next wake up feeling negative, hopeless, and unloving. Write this letter when you are feeling positive. What do you want to say to yourself on those hopeless days, so that the mere reading of this will trigger you back into positive thinking and restore love. Place this letter under your pillow for just such a day if it ever comes again.

DAY 37

Elephant Belief

I AM NOT SAFE TO FEEL ALL THAT I FEEL.

Today I went for an ultrasound and the man performing it seemed rude, cold, and clinical. I was not happy. I left feeling negatively affected, slightly disturbed, and unable to clear it. I reasoned with myself that I am strong and need not be affected, or perhaps should have expressed how I was feeling at the time. I wanted to call up and complain about him, to let the organization know how I was feeling, to let him know how I felt. I could feel anger stirring in me, as the victim part of myself came to the forefront. There was nothing I could do, I told myself, to make this right in me. Goodness, how do people survive more traumatic events, I asked myself?

All of a sudden the answer came to me. I was angry with myself. For what? Not speaking up? No. I was angry at myself for not acknowledging myself, my feelings, and my reaction. All I ever have to do is feel what I feel, not justify it, sort it out, or convince myself to get over it. These are the sorts of responses we give to each other and no doubt what were given to me as a child. I just need to feel upset, degraded, angry, and not have to put on a pretense to the contrary. Eventually these feelings will pass.

I sometimes think the pain of feeling my emotions will kill me, but actually it is denying them that slowly leads to my demise. I am designed to feel, not designed to suppress, deny, and avoid my true feelings.

My parents taught me that being in control of my emotions (i.e., suppressing how I really feel and being brave) means I am strong. This isn't being strong at all. This is being weak. Showing who I really am, first through my emotions, is real strength. In doing this I am transparent, honest, and real. This inner strength gives me the energy and vitality I need to transform myself and inspire others to do the same.

In regards to weight, fat is a natural result of not feeling my true emotions, because when I suppress my emotions, what I am actually doing is hiding them in myself—in the fat, the safest and surest insulator available to my body.

The solution to EVERY single conceivable problem in my life is through my feelings!

I got shivers down my spine as I suddenly had this realization. This one thing I try to avoid at all costs leads me to instead adopt an avoidance vice. Be it smoking, eating, overexercising, gambling, drinking, or something else—for each of us it may be different, but the reason is the same.

In order to heal physically, know the answers to my questions, resolve conflicts, and motivate myself, all I need to do is accept what I'm feeling and feel it fully.

Every time I avoid any negative emotion I give it permission to fester and reveal itself somewhere else in my life and body. Avoiding how I feel physically, emotionally, and mentally is like telling myself to shut up, and that I am not important.

I know now my aim in life was never to be healed or even to grow. I arrived here and stay all of life as learned, healed, and whole. What I am really here for is to be my authentic self. Being this means sharing my joy and insights. It means expressing *all* that I feel with myself. It means following my heart's desire even if it doesn't seem logical to me right now. It means being myself, showing love and kindness, and being forgiving to myself. It means loving unconditionally, while knowing it is impossible for my heart to ever break.

This is living my authentic life. I believe this is the reason and the only reason I was born into a human body and a human existence. Following this credo means I naturally heal and grow beyond the human conditioning that has caused me to forget how perfect I am, just as I am.

Angel Belief

I AM SAFE TO FEEL ALL OF MY EMOTIONS, AND IN DOING SO SET MYSELF FREE TO BE ME.

From Elephant to Angel Action

What emotions or feelings do you consider off limits to you? What emotions in yourself do you try to avoid feeling—anger, shame, guilt, resentment? Take the lid off these emotions today. Give yourself permission to feel EVERYTHING, even if only for today, and notice how this affects you, your day, and your reactions to other things and people around you. Is expressing your true feelings to yourself better or worse? Decide to do this as often as possible.

DAY 38

Elephant Belief

I STILL DON'T TRUST MYSELF TO EAT ANYTHING I WANT.

I'm having so much fun eating anything I want any time I want. It impresses on me today how individual our eating choices really are. I think most people would be surprised at what they would choose to eat each day, given the freedom to do so. I think our eating choices are just as unique and changeable as we are.

I find myself having days where I am eating a lot of fruit all day long and not much else until dinner. This is what I genuinely want to eat so I do. I feel free and alive and so full of energy. Of course the old me would never have allowed such a thing, particularly now when all the fitness and weight-loss gurus are saying no fruit (or very little) to lose weight. Magically when I begin following my own daily diet, I'm amazed by how thin I look almost immediately and the many compliments received about how slim I have become. The scales don't agree with this, but then who cares. I'm over scales. I don't really know what they are measuring, particularly since muscle weighs more than fat. I pick it up today and throw it out, literally, in the garbage!

I don't know what I will eat tomorrow or the day after, but this is not my concern because at this very minute I am free to eat as I please. I find that suddenly I am not thinking about food all day long, and my day is full of so much more to do other than just food purchasing, preparation, and cleaning up. I recall the horrified looks on student faces during my Elephants and Angels workshop when I would suggest to them, *"What if every time you think about food it has exactly the same effect as really eating it? How much more food are you really eating in a day?"*

You're better off eating real food than thinking about food all day long!

I remind myself today that I am safe to really eat food, rather than think about it all day and feel deprived. With each passing day I am trusting myself to eat anything I want.

I KNOW THAT WHEN I SET MYSELF FREE TO EAT AS I PLEASE, MY OWN UNIQUE WAY OF EATING DAY BY DAY WILL EMERGE.

From Elephant to Angel Action

Set your intention to eat whatever you genuinely want to eat. Follow your body, follow your inner urges, without judgment and without worry. All food is equal, so what do you want to eat?

DAY 39

Elephant Belief

I AM UNABLE TO CHANGE MY
NEGATIVE THOUGHTS.

I can easily transform my negative thoughts and emotions when I choose to.

The first step is to feel what I am feeling. I make no apology for it and this will minimize my taking it out on other people. I have noticed that, when I own my feelings, I grow stronger. I realize that, as uncomfortable as it is for me at the time, I survive. As I have grown more and more comfortable with this form of pain, I have also become better able to identify the true cause of my negative feelings.

The second step is for me to know it was something I was thinking earlier in the day or week that contributed to my negative thoughts and it will have been **about myself**. Even though I can think it is other people to blame, ultimately it is the negative thoughts that I have about myself that bring me down the most and create more negative thoughts. External things may have contributed but it is always a self-judgment that takes away my happiness and joy.

I can easily blame other people, my life situation, a lack of money, opportunity, or luck, but at the end of the day, the only person I am blaming for these things not being good enough is myself. I am not good enough. There will be a million things in a day that I "could" have done or "should" have done differently. I get angry, guilty, resentful, sad, and disappointed in *myself*. I always recognize that if someone is walking around in negative emotions, projecting these out to the world, they are really feeling this way about themselves.

This self-judgment is not going to get me anywhere, period. So long as I stay in this self-judgmental thinking, I'm sinking fast in quicksand, and it is a vicious cycle because it only gives me cause to hate myself even more.

Any negative judgment of myself is a condemnation to continue failing. Recognizing this is crucial.

I know I could easily say to myself, *"But look at my body—I'm fat—it's all my fault.*

Of course I deserve to feel bad about myself because I created it." Yet with this attitude I will only get fatter because I believe I have failed and don't deserve to be thin.

I am partway through my eighty-one days and I'm not getting thinner, and I'm angry with this silly approach to weight loss, but I know I am really only angry with myself and my body! Do I still believe there is something wrong with my body? Well, the only thing wrong with me is my thoughts, which are out of alignment with the real truth of me, which is love, perfection, and wholeness.

So the third step is to consciously choose to bring my focus and attention back to love and acceptance of myself. The truth is, I didn't put on ten pounds this week because of all the chocolate I ate, but because of the thoughts I had. That's why this change has to be a gradual one and in some ways a lifelong one. The rest of the world out there won't be thinking like me when I am done with this process, and they will try to brainwash me back to the negative approach because it makes sense to their minds. Not me! I am on a path to changing my consciousness for good. I will stay strong and focused, as I am already partway there. I just keep forgetting sometimes, and this book is here to keep reminding me until I can fully remember on my own.

Interestingly, the moment I turn off self-judgment and criticism, I also turn off all the "shoulds" in my head. And as I do what I really want to do, eat, and be, I suddenly become crystal clear. This is what I am on Earth to do—to be my authentic self.

Can I add, my body is not interested in my interpretation of it being fat, thin, or something in between. It wants to feel healthy, peaceful, and loved. It will go to the weight it's supposed to be and not the one my mind thinks it should be. So I will stop critiquing it and start focusing on feeling comfortable in my body, and then I know my body will start feeling comfortable in me.

Angel Belief

I CAN EASILY TRANSFORM MY NEGATIVE BELIEFS INTO NEW AND POSITIVE ONES AND I ALLOW THIS TO TRANSFORM MY LIFE.

From Elephant to Angel Action

Try this three-step process today if you find yourself feeling or thinking negatively:

Step 1:   Feel what you are feeling.

Step 2:   What negative self-judgment were you thinking about yourself earlier in the day or even yesterday or last week?

Step 3:   Consciously choose to bring your focus and attention back to love and acceptance of yourself. Write or think of all the things about yourself that you are grateful for. Forgive yourself for all the negativity. It was never real to begin with. It was only a perception, a thought—and a thought can be changed.

DAY 40

Elephant Belief

I HAVE LOTS OF FEARS THAT CONTROL MY LIFE.

I recognize today that the fight I have been carrying out has never been with my body. The fight is with my fear. I've been fighting with fear and my choice of either running from it or fighting with it. This is the fight my body and mind keep playing out. My solution, therefore, is to stop fighting. I will never win the fight. I realize that fear doesn't have to be overcome, just recognized. When I recognize the fears I have about anything, I can think the fear out of my life. Any conflict, injury, body resistance is always because of the fear associated with it. I only make "wrong" decisions, in retrospect, when there is fear motivating me.

There is nothing wrong with my body except the fear. I no longer need to fear becoming overweight. I no longer need to fear food. I no longer have to fear other people's judgments of me. I no longer need to fear myself. I need to begin where I am, with who I am today, and in this way I will allow a new doorway to open to myself to be even better. Whatever I reject today, stays and digs its heels in, being even harder to remove from my life tomorrow.

Fear lives in the amygdala gland of the brain and comes from past experiences. I have had so many clients over the years who have feared getting sick with a particular illness, and then have returned, sometimes years later, with the very illness they feared. Did they develop this illness because they feared it, or were they fearing it because they could sense they would eventually have it? It is an interesting question, but I still believe it is the former. I believe our thinking attracts into our life the very thing we fear.

Angel Belief

I RELEASE ALL OF MY FEARS.
I AM SAFE AND SECURE.
MY FUTURE IS SAFE AND SECURE.

From Elephant to Angel Action

Agree to release all fear in you today. Close your eyes and imagine a pink soothing light shining on the amygdala gland of your brain, cleaning away old fears accumulated there that stand in the way of being all that you came here to be. Wait patiently until this feels complete and remember to give thanks! Breathe deeply.

DAY 41

I CAN'T MEDITATE OR FAST.
THAT'S TOO HARD FOR ME.

I notice a lot of people have resistance to meditation, and I used to be very much the same when I started. I have come to realize that this resistance is due to the fact that meditation can bring up repressed fears, self-judgments, and negative emotions. I used to wonder why after meditating I felt worse than before. Sometimes I would be crystal clear and full of love during my meditation, and would find when I emerged from it, that I was really angry and very snappy at my children. It was then I realized meditation isn't just a feel good thing to tick off the list. Just like anything else that challenges me, it is there to show me my self-perceived weaknesses so I can overcome them and move past them.

I believe a healthy level of challenge is a crucial and essential part of life because it reveals the still unloved parts of myself. When I remember this, I start enjoying meditation, exercise, and other challenges in my life. Challenges exist for me to grow through them, not to limit me. There is always a way through any challenge and it involves loving and believing in myself.

Is meditation a "must do?" No, nothing is, but having experienced the tremendous benefits of meditation on my health, mind, and body, I know that even a little meditation is worth a lot. I recommend any form of meditation, whether it be a silent mode or an active mode. I do not believe you need to be quite so prescriptive about how often to do it, but doing it will give amazing results at changing beliefs and harmonizing emotions. I find when I am struggling with any activity, be it meditation or exercise, it is usually because I am judging myself, comparing myself to others, or forcing myself to do the activity when I do not really want to on that particular day. But I patiently persist when I feel positive about it again and it begins to pay off.

I also find the act of fasting to be a beneficial practice, now and again. Some people fast regularly, whether for a day or longer. Some people do fasts where they can still have juices or other minimal foods, while others fast by eating no food at all. Fasting has been shown to have tremendously positive effects on the body for health reasons and beyond. Calorie restriction is linked with higher longevity rates.

A method of fasting that I particularly enjoy doing now and again to reset my appetite or cleanse during the spring time is a method called Pi Gu Fasting. I imagine I am eating and drinking the food and beverage I am about to really eat before I actually eat it. So for example, if I am about to eat pizza, I take a few minutes to imagine eating it first in my mind. What is the purpose of this? Doing this will make me feel more satisfied after having eaten, and I rarely overeat when doing this technique. You see, I eat with my mind first, and then with my mouth. It is a really useful technique! It can also be used in place of food and water altogether. You won't feel hungry or deprived. It's amazingly effective.

Angel Belief

I SEE THE BENEFIT IN MEDITATING AND COMMIT TO SUCH PRACTICES FOR MY HIGHEST HEALING.

From Elephant to Angel Action

Spend just five minutes today in a meditative practice. Allow this meditation to be done by yourself, no music, no guidance—just you and a silent space for five tiny minutes. In this five minutes focus your attention on breathing into your heart space, followed by breathing into your sacral chakra, just below your navel. Imagine as you breathe that on the inhale all sickness and negativity is collecting in your body at the point you are breathing into. As you exhale, breathe this negativity and sickness out of your body through your mouth. Then breathe in again, taking in fresh, vibrant energy into your body.

Try Pi Gu Fasting with at least one of your meals today, as I described above. Aim to do this with the meal time that you normally eat the most, and see what difference it makes to how you eat and feel. You can still eat your food afterward.

DAY 42

REST DAY

Today is a day of rest. I spend the day praising my middle torso—the stomach, which is the place of digestion and creation, and all the organs inside me that work so hard. I love and acknowledge them. They love me and I choose to love them back. I imagine smiling at them on this day and everyday. In fact I wake up each morning and the first thing I do before getting out of bed is to smile to my internal organs, awakening them and energizing them. Smiling at the organs each morning is an ancient Chinese method of awakening the organs and keeping them healthy. I also give thanks on this day for being human, and remind myself that as I love my body, it loves me in return.

Extra weight on the stomach represents creativity waiting to be birthed. Extra weight on the backside represents trouble letting go of the past, and fat around the midsection often affectionately called the 'tire' represents feeling held back either by others or by life. It also represents a desire to express so much, and to give so much more, but feeling limited to do so. I use the A.N.G.E.L process to remove these limitations today freeing myself to change.

DAY 43

Elephant Belief

I KEEP MY WEIGHT DOWN BECAUSE I EXERCISE REGULARLY AND EAT HEALTHY FOOD.

I'm not going to lie and pretend that I wrote this book because I get up every morning and eat chocolate cake, hamburgers, and fries. I don't. I eat exceptionally healthily most of the time, but I do eat at least ten times a day or more, way more that I am "supposed" to! I exercise regularly, meditate when I can, and practice martial arts and Qi Gong a few times each week.

Now, perhaps you might ask what right I have to tell you how to lose weight eating anything you want, while not appearing to do this myself. However, I believe doing those things are not what keep me slim. Most other people that exercise or eat well think this is what ensures they remain slim. I do not personally believe this. I believe it is always about how people think and their attitude—this is why they're thin. I know women who exercise a great deal at a very high intensity and eat very little and are still what might be considered over the healthy weight range. They may not believe in themselves or have other negative beliefs that are limiting their weight. I have a close friend that eats pastries like they're going out of fashion and sits around all day. She's really thin and this is because her self-esteem is really high.

So I'm a great advocate for eating well, exercising, and meditating because these things help break through my negative thinking and set me free. I do these things because they are pure fun for me, and fun is my number one most important value. If I do notice I am genuinely putting on weight, instead of asking, *"What have I been eating,"* I ask myself, *"What have I been thinking?"*

Angel Belief

EATING MORE NATURALLY BASED FOODS AND EXERCISING ARE WONDERFUL PRACTICES TO DO FOR HEALTH, BUT IT IS ALWAYS MY THINKING THAT KEEPS ME THIN.

From Elephant to Angel Action

Catch yourself every time you have a negative thought about yourself today and remind yourself: *"It is not what I eat that makes me gain weight, it is what I think."* Promise yourself that you are worth thinking positive thoughts about. Choose to eat healthy food and exercise because it is fun and helps you grow as a person, and not just to keep you thin.

DAY 44

Elephant Belief

I DON'T THINK ANY OF THIS WORK IS CHANGING MY CORE BELIEFS ABOUT FOOD AND MY BODY. I FEEL THE SAME.

Through my work with clients over the years I have observed that beliefs live in the heart center and are made up of *thoughts* from the higher chakras combined with *feelings* from the lower chakras. Together, our thoughts and feelings based on past events fuse together at the heart chakra to create a true and lasting belief.

Beliefs guide our entire life. We are often not aware of our beliefs consciously as they live in the subconscious mind. They reveal themselves through our actions, the words that come out of our mouths, and especially the ways we react to things. We may think we believe one thing, but our actions and reactions reveal the beliefs we are truly ruled by.

To change old beliefs, therefore, I need to create new thoughts and new feelings within myself and maintain them long enough for them to turn into knowing. A knowing within me is even stronger than a belief and resides in the unconscious mind, which regulates heart beat, breath, and metabolism. It is the automatic part of us all. The unconscious mind is the seat of the intuition, the place where inspiration is born.

Knowing is the concrete level of belief.

In order to be able to truly lose weight while eating anything I desire, I must actually know this is both possible and know that I can achieve it. I may believe that for this to happen I need to unearth and discover all of the current beliefs I have about food, fat, thinness, gaining weight, losing weight, self-esteem, self-love, boundaries with others, judgment, and change. Basically all the beliefs I have about me!

While this is one approach, and I am partially doing this through my eighty-one days of exploration, there is also a much easier way. This way involves working with energy. In Chinese medicine, there is a belief that if you tap into the master's energy, then you can do the extraordinary healing that he or she can do. It is all about utilizing the energy correctly. When I work on clients I release the most difficult past events, change more than a handful of limiting beliefs, and have the client feeling light, balanced, and free all in a one-hour session. Using energy principles to release old habitual beliefs that are limiting people is very easy and quick. I can move energy very efficiently and release old patterns in a fraction of the time compared to doing it the way I was formally trained in psychology. The energy way is powerful and so efficient!

This book and each of the days is not simply about the words. Hidden within the words are the frequency of change, the frequency of what I believe about myself and others, and the frequency of love and inner healing. The change is going to occur in whoever reads this book.

In some ways the less you try to make it happen, the more likely it will. This is because the change is encrypted at the energetic level and being the master that has written this book in this instance, whoever is led to follow my lead will succeed because I have succeeded. I believe when we read any book, it's never really about the words or even the messages, but always about the energy of the writer to whom we are drawn.

Angel Belief

I AM CHANGING. I CAN FEEL IT.
I AM CHANGING AT THE VERY CELLULAR
LEVEL OF MY BEING. I EMBRACE NEW BELIEFS
ABOUT LIFE AND MYSELF.

From Elephant to Angel Action

Close your eyes right now and allow the highest wisdom within you to take your old self-limiting beliefs away. Imagine if it helps that you are lying on my very own treatment table receiving a healing. Allow yourself to be rebalanced in all ways.

Allow your nervous system to be balanced, your hormones, and your spleen, which are all related to stress and anxiety. If these organs are not working properly, they turn any food into fat instead of muscle.

DAY 45

Elephant Belief

I CAN'T BE HONEST ABOUT HOW I REALLY FEEL AND I CANNOT EVER BE TOTALLY HEALED.

I want so much to express how I am feeling today. I woke up this morning with questions and turmoil in my mind and instantly noticed the familiar pain and numbing in the right side of my body which I have been experiencing on and off for the past year. It suddenly returned after months of it just not being an issue anymore. *"Wow,"* I thought, *"my body really does reflect my thoughts."* The more I truly understand this law of the universe, the quicker my thoughts reflect through my body as seeming illness or imbalance. My body really is mirroring my thoughts.

I am so scared to feel what I feel. I was taught this from a young age. I am so scared that if I follow my dreams, leave the relationships that drain me, start something new, that I might end up making the wrong choice—so I eat instead. I eat to cover my gut feelings and to numb myself. To be addicted to food is an addiction to avoidance—an avoidance of how I feel. When I gain weight it is to avoid myself. I hide my real self under layers of fat because it just feels easier that way. It hurts too much to reveal it. It hurts too much to know I have lived, at times, a powerless life and not valued myself. It is so much easier to expect the things I do not give myself to come from others instead. I keep limiting the good I allow myself to gain through my own self-love and acceptance.

Today it's time for me to give myself permission to feel again. When I woke up this morning with the right side of my body in pain and inflammation, my thoughts were saying, *"Go back to work in the clinic. It's good money, you love working with people. You cannot make a good living as an author. Go back to work. It is good work and you are safe there. You are loved and successful there."* But my true feelings kept saying, *"No more! As good and easy as it is, I don't want to go back."* The truth is, if I were dying tomorrow, I would feel that I had not achieved everything that I had come to do.

My mind is constantly battling with my heart. While it may seem logical and practical for me to go back to seeing clients, my heart wants more. To stop seeing clients in person was a difficult decision for me to make, as I really did love it, and yet I knew it was time for me to grow further. What I am stepping into next in my life may appear scary, difficult, and unattainable even, but so long as I deny the true yearnings of my heart, I deny me, and **then I eat**. I eat to escape the truth, to deny my true inner yearnings, and to avoid being my true self.

Today I listen to my feelings, and I feel safe enough to voice them. When I am feeling this way, I do not choose whether to listen to my head or my heart. I ignore them both actually, because so long as they are battling each other, I will get hurt if I get involved. Instead I allow them to battle it out, without the observer in me joining in, and I do something on those days that is nurturing and fun instead. I wait it out. No decision can yet be made and to try to will only make me suffer. My head and heart will sort it out, and so long as I am consciously out of the way, I know my heart will always win. It always does when I just get out of its way.

When the battle is done, I will know. I will feel safe, sure, and excited again. I will follow my heart and I will be the author I know I have come to be. Today, as I finally follow my heart and finally begin being and doing what I have come to be and do, no matter how scary it may be, then any remaining food issues just disappear on their own. The health symptoms with which I awoke have now disappeared! No medication or treatment of any kind. I do not need them anymore to teach me or to guide me. I know what my body was trying to tell me and I have understood.

Angel Belief

I LISTEN TO MY BODY AND FEELINGS AS A GUIDE TO MY INNER SELF. AS I FOLLOW MY INNER GUIDANCE ALL DISEASE DISAPPEARS.

From Elephant to Angel Action

Pay attention to how your body is feeling today in each and every circumstance you find yourself in. Pay attention to your emotions. At the end of the day, write a list in your journal of the things in your life you love to do and the things you hate doing. Be honest! No one is going to see this list other than you. Be careful you are not tricking yourself. Be guided by your feelings in the here and now, just like my feeling of *"I don't want to see clients anymore."* It doesn't mean I will always feel this way. No feeling is ever wrong!

Write your list based on what you feel today, right now. You are permitted to write another list tomorrow that contradicts this one. Be truthful. Now decide to begin from this day forth to act on this list. You do not need to know how. You only need to set the intent to have few, if any, things in any of your days that you hate, and lots of things in your days that you love.

DAY 46

Elephant Belief

I OFTEN FEEL GUILT AND SHAME AND FEED ON OTHERS' GUILT AND SHAME.

I know within myself when I behave unkindly to myself or others. When I am honest during those times, then I have the ability to forgive myself and move along. This also empowers me to be kinder in future. A lot of the time, however, I just end up feeling guilty or shameful instead.

Shame and guilt are the lowest vibrational emotions that can be felt. Hence, when my self-esteem is low, I will often judge other people, causing them to feel guilty or shameful and then I will feed on these emotions, feeling better about myself. Somehow if someone else feels less than me, this can make me feel better. But it's a really poor way to feel better about myself. In reality, my high is short lived, as putting someone else down only brings me down with them.

Many of us raise our children through shame and guilt. I know I do sometimes. It simply works. I was mostly raised this way. I am very guilty of feeling guilt all of the time. Guilt is my Achilles' heel. I use guilt to motivate myself to do the right things, and to punish other people when they do not do the right things. I blame other people for all sorts of things and then feel guilty for doing so. I'm caught in a cycle of pain, fueled by guilt and shame. I'm also ashamed that as I was writing this, I just ate half of the leftover chocolate pudding from last night. It's a good thing calories aren't real, and all food is neutral! But I still feel guilty.

I remind myself the solution to my affliction is love and forgiveness. I need to forgive myself for my less than kind behaviors and thoughts. And what if I hurt others? Can I say sorry without feeling guilty, bad about myself, or needing to justify myself? Yes, of course I can. When I say sorry without experiencing these negative emotions, then I am genuinely sorry. In this case, I am sorry not to escape my own guilt, but because I genuinely care about others.

My vibration of wellness is not affected by what happens to me in life, how I am treated by others, or even how I treat myself. My vibration of health and well-being is only ever defined by *my perception* and response to myself, others, and external events. The plain and simple truth is *I choose* this reaction, in each and every moment of my life. The more unconscious and unaware I am, the more unconscious my choices are. That is why the more aware I become, the more freedom I have to choose my responses consciously. I gain the ability to free myself of my own self-condemnation through the conscious act of self-forgiveness. Each time I forgive myself I grow stronger and clearer and less likely to act in ways that require forgiveness at all.

Today I proclaim that I love and forgive myself for all unkind behavior and thinking I have had toward myself and others. In fact I will even forgive myself on behalf of others that do not understand enough to forgive me yet. My own forgiveness is what really counts. Boy, do I feel better already!

Angel Belief

I RELEASE GUILT AND SHAME AND FORGIVE MYSELF FOR ALL THAT I SAY AND DO TO MYSELF AND OTHERS.

From Elephant to Angel Action

As you move through your day, notice how many times you think unkind thoughts about yourself or others, and instantly state to yourself, *"I forgive myself."* Do this over and over again throughout your day. You may be surprised by how many negative thoughts, perceptions, and reactions you actually have through the day. Probably many. It doesn't matter how many, just keep forgiving yourself over and over again as required. Notice by the end of the day how you feel within yourself compared to other days where you do not carry out this exercise. Any guilt or shame-filled emotions can be forgiven in you right now. It is the best way for you to move forward. There is nothing in this world that you can do to render yourself unforgivable, and I mean nothing.

The only person's forgiveness that you need is your own.

DAY 47

Elephant Belief

I AM FAT AND BLOATED.

I woke up today feeling fat and bloated. The mirror told me the same thing. Even my clothes seemed to agree, feeling snugger than usual. Once upon a time I would have tried to make myself feel better by eating everything I could get my hands on. Funny, because now technically I can do this without gaining weight and yet I don't really want to anymore.

I give myself some time for self-reflection to find the real answer to what is going on in my body. I discover that when I am feeling and even looking this way, my energy is beginning to go inward. I am drawing away from the outer world to inner solitude. My bloated stomach says to the world, *"Stay away! It is my time just for me."* Interesting. My body also tells me that I do not need to panic, as nothing has gone wrong in my body. Instead, when I wake up feeling fat for no apparent reason, my body is preparing to birth a brand new creative endeavor. Often women can find this happens around the time of their menses, as this too is the time of drawing inward preparing for what could potentially be a time of creation. Creation is a wondrous thing, and it does require that we shut the world out and hibernate. It is a time to be with myself, the people I love, and to give to myself, before once again going out into the world and sharing.

Anita Johnston PhD, in her wonderful book *Eating in the Light of the Moon*, refers to women often experiencing "fat attack" days. These are days when we wake up feeling inexplicably fatter, but realistically we could not possibly have gained that much weight overnight. Sometimes we even experience this feeling in the course of a day. A "fat attack" comes on suddenly and is intense in nature. Anita explains that a "fat attack" is usually a signal of a hidden feeling within that is not being acknowledged.

I decide that from now on when I wake up feeling this way I will celebrate instead of lament, as I have been given permission to have a lazy day and just have fun without pressuring or expecting anything from myself. Sure, I will probably eat lots of sugar on days such as this, but I trust my body will go right back to normal again quickly. I allow myself the time and space to bring up whatever deep within me may be troubling me. These days are my days. Time for me, to be with me.

Angel Belief

I AM BEAUTIFUL JUST AS I AM EACH AND EVERY DAY. I NURTURE MYSELF AT ALL TIMES AND ALLOW MY TRUTH AND CREATIVITY TO BE REVEALED.

From Elephant to Angel Action

Imagine today you are having a "fat attack" day. Spend the day listening to your deeper yearnings. This is not a day to escape from or to blame yourself. Listen to your internal messages, body cues, and feelings. Allow the spiritual guidance from within you to inform you. Be with yourself rather than rushing around in the external world, avoiding yourself.

Today is a day to find the true you hidden under all of the false agreements you have made with yourself and society. Fat attack days are not an attack at all, but rather an opportunity to surrender. On this day, a unique opportunity is presented to you to take your fears, overwhelming emotions, internal conflicts, and limiting beliefs and hand them over to a higher power, allowing these things to be resolved by the highest part within your self. Reframe today so that you realize that extra fat has not suddenly attacked you from somewhere external to you. Instead, this fat has come from within you and is waiting to be released and set free. You do not require it anymore. Celebrate this day and let it go with joy and gratitude.

DAY 48

Elephant Belief

I AM NOT ALLOWED TO EXPRESS MY TRUE SELF AROUND OTHER PEOPLE.

It can be hard to be me some days. At least this is how I feel today. It seems the more comfortable I am in my own skin and living my truth, the more I upset or offend the people around me. I have done this too many times to even list. A friend whose party I attended recently mentioned afterward that I had offended many people at the party. She went on to say that she could tell I liked to upset people on purpose! I was a little shocked. Expressing my opinion was regarded by others as a judgment toward them or simply wrong of me.

I thought about this for some time and came to the conclusion that I will not feel responsible for other people's reactions to me being myself, or stop speaking my truth. My friend felt uncomfortable when I stated truths that challenged her and others emotionally. However, I can have compassion for her in this and make an extra effort to keep my opinions and feelings to myself around her. This is not lying to myself or pretending. This is being mindful of others. I can own my thoughts and feelings without always sharing them.

The most important thing is that I am always being honest and present within myself and to myself.

I can choose to no longer get upset about other people's opinions of me and I do not need to be upset with myself for having done something wrong. All I need to do is be accepting of myself. I need not be defined by other people's judgments of me. My choices today are what define me. One day when the whole world feels the same way, we can all happily express everything and we will not be perceived to judge or be judged. We will all know and understand that full expression is an absolute joy and part of the freedom of life. Why is this a relevant learning for me today around food and my body? Because every time somebody makes a negative judgment of me, I often shut down, feel bad, and eat! Not anymore.

Awareness is setting me free!

I EXPRESS MY FEELINGS AND THOUGHTS FREELY AND CHOOSE WITH DISCERNMENT WHEN TO DO THIS AROUND OTHER PEOPLE.

From Elephant to Angel Action

Become aware on this day of all the times you are not being your true self. Notice how many times you lie to others today. Perhaps you tell a friend she looks nice in what she's wearing, but you do not really mean it. Perhaps you say to your partner that you love the dinner that is prepared when you really would have loved to be eating something else. Perhaps you tell your children you love taking caring of them when you would really rather be at the spa today. Notice the lies you constantly tell yourself.

Noticing is the beginning of realizing that you are rarely being your true self, particularly around others. As you do this today, ask yourself, *"Can I actually say the truth in this situation?"* You might be surprised how often the answer is "yes." The more you begin to be honest instead of keeping the peace with others, the more people will respect you and be given permission to be the same. Remember the only person you need to tell the truth to is yourself.

DAY 49

REST DAY

Today I allow myself to rest and to revel in the excitement and freedom to eat whatever I like whenever I like. My daughter this morning said to me, *"I'm the luckiest girl in the world because I'm the only person I know that's allowed to eat ice cream for breakfast."* Sometimes indeed she does, and she loves it and then moves on to apples and carrots easily and effortlessly without judgment! She feels free and loves her body and I want to have this same child-like attitude. I have gratitude today just like my daughter, and give myself permission to be just as free.

Today I eat whatever I really genuinely want for breakfast, lunch, dinner, and in between, no matter what it is. I give thanks for my taste buds and gratitude for having so many choices available to me. I am so lucky! Food is a wonderful adventure to wake up to each and every day, so I give thanks for this over and over again.

DAY 50

Elephant Belief

I HAVE PUT ON WEIGHT BECAUSE I HAVEN'T BEEN EXERCISING!

Today was a reminder for me to be careful of good old self-judgment sneaking back in when I'm not aware. I guess sometimes it feels like I've been there and done that so it must be gone now . . . FOREVER. The reminder is that so long as I'm human, there will often be a tendency to return to my old ways of thinking because they exist in my subconscious mind. When I catch these old thoughts returning, however, I will remember more easily and let them go again and again, until eventually they have nowhere to return from.

What happened to teach me this important lesson today? I went to the gym after not having gone at all for a week. My intent in going was pure at the time; that is, I was there for joy and fun. I felt like having a work out and everything seemed to support this as my schedule cleared up and I had a couple of hours all to myself. As I was in the aerobics room by myself, doing some boxing and weights, I suddenly looked at myself in the mirror and briefly heard my mind think, *"Gee, I look fat!."* I continued without paying too much notice, after all my mind throws around all kinds of thoughts in a day. As I continued to work out, I found myself in disbelief at how much weight I felt I had gained in a week of no exercise. Sure I was eating whatever I wanted, but I always did lately and had not gained any weight.

I finished my workout and went home. I ended up spending the rest of the day eating my way through house and home. At first I felt fine about doing this, but then I realized that my eating behavior on this occasion was not just me eating extra from a place of love and joy, but a self-punishing kind of eating. I then became aware of my voice of self-judgment stating I just ate things that were bad! I instantly recognized what had led to my self-loathing behavior and a backward slide in my thinking. It was my scathing perception of myself in the mirror earlier in the day. I laughed at myself in an instant and spent the rest of the day back in the natural flow of my body rather than drowning in the unrelenting self-judgment I had given myself earlier. I forgave myself instantly. Whether it was true I had gained weight or not was not the point. If I had, I trust that my body would correct this, but it can never correct my self-judgment. My judgment would only take me back to a space of punishing myself further.

Funnily enough, the very next day at the gym, one of the trainers complimented me on how I had lost weight over the last week! How ironic, given my own perception only a day earlier and an afternoon of nonstop eating. She emphatically let me know that sometimes the body loses weight when we take a rest and do not exercise for a week, because the body recovers properly from too much movement. What a giant lesson in releasing self-judgment and not always believing my critical self-perception.

Angel Belief

I TRUST MY BODY TO MAINTAIN ITS NATURAL WEIGHT DESPITE NOT EXERCISING. I REMIND MYSELF TO MOVE FOR JOY AND ENERGY RATHER THAN TO LOSE WEIGHT.

From Elephant to Angel Action

Do you partake in a form of movement just for fun and joy? Commit today to find a form of movement that you do from a place of love and joy rather than to keep thin. Exercising to keep thin is a fear-based approach and can lead to physical injury and limitation. Exercising for joy keeps you thin naturally, but more importantly lets your body know it is loved. You feel healthier as a result. If you already have a form of exercise that you do every week, pay attention as to what your motivation is.

Decide today: *"I move for the joy and energy this gives me. I am naturally thin without this movement. This movement feeds my soul as much as it energizes my body."*

DAY 51

IT IS NOT MY FAULT I HAVE EATING ISSUES. IT IS OTHER PEOPLE'S FAULT.

Today I was reflecting how many of my food issues stem from my mother and father. They use food as a reward, and I often find myself rewarding myself through food. Food was not to be wasted when I was little and one of my earliest memories was my mother shoveling food into her mouth every chance she got. In fact, I rarely remember her not eating. Knowing my mother, she was probably shoveling food into my mouth, too! The other thing I remember about my mother is, if she wasn't eating continuously, she was on the latest diet. Even today, when I visit my mother and father, their number one obsession and favorite topic of conversation is how to lose weight and their latest method for doing so. They are constantly complaining about their weight and obsessed with food and eating.

It is easy for me to blame them for my food issues, but blaming them is no solution for how I eat today and no way to transform myself in this regard. So long as I harbor any resentment toward them and any others that showed me unloving ways to relate to food, I will always be filling myself with more food to cover up the gaping hole within myself. Through letting it all go and forgiving these people, I set myself free for a new beginning, recognizing that these learnings have made me strong and educated. In fact if I did not have these experiences, I would not even be here now sharing my insights with others. My new mantra is *"accept, accept, accept"* and *"forgive, forgive, forgive."* Accepting and forgiving life and all the people and events within it gives me the most immense transformational power. I find myself rising above all events. I have great clarity, no stress, and I have access to the most creative solutions to problems that arise from time to time. As I change and forgive, I give other people permission to do the same.

Angel Belief

I FORGIVE AND RELEASE ALL THE PEOPLE WHO PLAYED A PART IN INFLUENCING MY DECISIONS AROUND FOOD. I SET MYSELF FREE.

From Elephant to Angel Action

Think of all the people that have influenced you in relation to food and in relation to how you feel about your body. Recognize that so long as you hold on to any resentment toward them you stay entrapped by their influence. They no longer exist in the here and now. In this moment you are free to be a new you and adopt a fresh way of relating to food and to yourself.

Today affirm: *"I accept and forgive all people who have influenced my relationship to food, to my body, and even to life itself in a seemingly negative way. I release them and in so doing release myself to be free."*

DAY 52

Elephant Belief

I FEEL I AM ABOUT TO GAIN WEIGHT
AND I AM POWERLESS TO STOP IT.

Over the years I have noticed that, just before I am about to begin gaining weight, I have felt what can only be described as a switch going off in my head. This probably sounds quite strange, but it really feels just like that, and when this happens I know that no matter what I do, I will now gain weight as a result. Well, today I caught what this switch actually is. I felt it occurring in my head, and using the medical intuitive abilities I now have, I watched to see what was happening in my own brain and body.

What was this magical switch-like thing? Well, to me it appeared to be my thalamus. The thalamus is a gland in the center of the brain that filters sensory information and regulates motor functions in the body. From my understanding, watching it in action rather than reading about it in books, it informs the hypothalamus as well as the amygdala gland. It informs lots of other parts of the body too, but these two connections where fascinating to me, given the role the hypothalamus has in regulating appetite and eating behavior and the role of the amygdala gland in relation to triggering subconscious fear.

When I asked my body for more information about the thalamus, it let me know that it is affected and "switched" off when my male-female balance and internal-external balance is thrown off within me. I was told that when my inner-outer authority and masculine-feminine balance is lost, my "switch" is turned to the negative. In other words, when I reject my inner voice and my inner feminine nature, which are based on feelings, intuition, and trust, I then rely more on the logical, controlled, masculine self and am influenced predominantly by the external world. It is important to use both the masculine and feminine parts of myself rather than either one or the other.

Anita Johnston PhD, in her book *Eating in the Light of the Moon*, supports this view, that disordered eating in women is a consequence of the masculine and feminine aspects being out of balance. She states, "Rather than trusting our bodies to inform us when we are in need of physical nourishment or stimulation, we follow elaborate diet plans and rigid exercise regimes."

My thalamus is responding to a decision I make that others know better than I do, and I need to do as others see best. When I think this way, I also decide that my feelings are best avoided because they could potentially cause an interference with my goals.

I love the way Anita Johnston goes on to say that, "When the masculine controls the feminine, there is a lot of action without meaning." She further explains that women try to make their bodies look masculine, losing their curvaceous natural form. We want flat stomachs and no hips, when this is not the natural design of the female body. Looking around at the gym, honestly, the fittest women to me look like men with long hair!

I accept all of this today and use my intent to correct the thalamus in my brain, allowing it to also reflect the feminine and internally based world. The outer world and masculine allure is hard for me to resist, but I recognize that it really doesn't serve me. It may always be my weakness, but from now on if I recognize that "switch" going off in my head, I will put it right again immediately.

One last question to myself: why does the thalamus potentially trigger weight gain? The answer comes effortlessly. The thalamus is triggered by emotional suppression, alerting the fat cells within my body that they will soon be needed to cocoon the ensuing emotions I am not expressing that need to be stored away safely. The female aspect of myself, however, always expresses, and the thalamus remains balanced.

Angel Belief

I CORRECT MY THALAMUS EASILY THROUGH MY INTENT AND BRING BALANCE BACK TO MY MASCULINE-FEMININE ASPECTS.

From Elephant to Angel Action

In your journal today, write what you perceive to be the weaknesses of males and the weaknesses of females. Use this exercise to reveal to you what you perceive as being undesirable in each of the two sexes.

Do you try to be too masculine? Do you embrace the feminine qualities of yourself (whether you are a male or a female) as we all have both within us?

Close your eyes and ask that pink light infuse your entire head, rebalancing your thalamus and bringing equality back within you. Breathe deeply and release. It is done.

DAY 53

Elephant Belief

I STILL CANNOT EAT ANYTHING I WANT AND LOSE WEIGHT.

I just finished running my first *Eat Like An Elephant Look Like An Angel* workshop. Hooray! It was such a major learning experience as I myself am still on this journey, and not yet complete in my own journey, at day fifty-three. I shared this with the workshop group. Honesty is one of my most important values and it was encouraging and refreshing to them to know that even though I am not quite there yet myself, I am making great progress. At this point in time, I can now eat anything I like and no longer gain weight, but am unsure how to lose weight.

Well, I was blown away in this workshop by how much the attendees taught me, rather than the other way around! I listened intently as one of the participants, who happened to sit directly next to me (as we all sat in a circle), told her story. She was overweight as a child and at some point decided that she wanted to lose weight. The amazing part of her story was, she lost the weight and has remained very thin ever since, but she never made a connection in her mind between weight loss and food reduction. In other words she never believed that in order to lose weight she had to stop eating certain foods, or eat less. Wow! She lost weight without changing what she ate. She made the decision and that was that. She was a living example of what I was professing, and had been this way ever since childhood. Not to mention that she was constantly eating at this workshop!

The second amazing occurrence at the workshop was a participant who literally made the quantum shift and changed her body as a result of this book's teachings. The day before the workshop she was shopping for a new pair of pants. Having tried on a size 14, she decided against buying them. The day after the workshop, just one day later, she went back to buy those pants after all and was indeed suddenly a size 12! May I add that even though the workshop was about eating anything you like and losing weight, most of the participants were very conscious of what they ate, and ate very little throughout the day. This particular participant, however, ate a great deal. She said of the workshop later, *"I really got it when you said that broccoli and chocolate are the same. Just energy. I made the mind shift."*

These two examples at my first workshop are giant proof that I need to continue on this path of changing my relationship to food forever. Proof that educating people about this new approach is important!

I have decided as a result that I can and will lose those last few pounds easily and effortlessly and do it just for me, without changing what I eat. Easy. If others can do it, I can too!

Angel Belief

I CAN EAT ANYTHING I WANT AND LOSE WEIGHT.

From Elephant to Angel Action

Think of someone you know that can eat whatever they want and never seem to gain weight. Write about them, describing how and what they eat. Now place yourself in the story, describing how you are the same. Describe yourself as if you can eat whatever you want with no consequence. Describe how not only can you maintain your weight eating whatever you like, but you can even lose weight. Go on to describe what you ate and how much weight you lost. Doing this exercise in written form is very powerful. Commit to reading this for three days and notice how you change in your ability to eat anything you like and actually lose weight.

DAY 54

Elephant Belief

I AM EASILY INFLUENCED BY OTHERS WHEN I EAT IN THEIR PRESENCE.

"Beware of eating with others!"

That was the sentence I suddenly heard clearly in my own mind. I knew what the message was alluding to. Sure, I am making wonderful progress in this journey, but when I eat with other people who are still influenced by external beliefs about food and weight, I become influenced by them and revert back to my old ways of thinking. Until my new beliefs grow deep and long-lasting roots, I am still vulnerable. I find other people's beliefs begin to make me question all I have worked toward.

I also observe my strange behavior at feeling better somehow when other people eat badly. As if their poor eating makes me better than they are. If I believe that all food is equal, why don't I yet project this belief to others, making them have the benefits that I get from this belief system?

I notice what else I think when I am eating with others, and find that I sometimes want to fit in, be part of the crowd, so I act as though I believe what they believe, rather than living by my own beliefs. At other times I tell people on purpose that I am writing this book in order to see how they react to the controversial claim this book makes. I am surprised and sometimes disheartened by the fact that they cannot grasp such a concept and even try to convince me about the importance of eating only healthy food and the latest fad diet they are planning to undertake.

I let it all go. I am not the group. I am an individual, and as I know and believe more and more in my own approach to eating, the only person I need to believe in is myself. I will march on, aware of myself in groups but always reaching back to my new intention to make this change for me.

Angel Belief

NO ONE CAN INFLUENCE MY BELIEFS ABOUT EATING. MY BELIEFS ARE MY OWN. I AM SAFE TO EAT AS I PLEASE.

From Elephant to Angel Action

As you progress through these changes notice how you relate to this new way of seeing food, particularly when you are around others. Does your family see food in the same way? Are you supported in this new way of being? Notice the weak links in your thinking where you allow yourself to be influenced by the media, friends, and other people. As you notice your own doubts still present, place your intent back on what this book is teaching you. Reaffirm the many benefits of being free around food. Remind yourself this journey is worth it. Today try to convince no one else other than the deepest part of yourself that this really is REAL and it is working for you.

DAY 55

Elephant Belief

IT IS EASIER FOR OTHER PEOPLE TO BELIEVE IN THEMSELVES, LOVE THEMSELVES AND EAT MORE NATURALLY BASED FOODS. THEIR LIFE IS EASY COMPARED TO MINE.

It is so easy to envy other people, especially those who seem to keep slim so effortlessly while I seem to have to slave away to maintain a slim figure. Every morning while dropping off my son at school I would notice a mom walking her child to school. She always looked the same to me, consistent, happy, and thin. I would notice her every day in envy, wondering how she managed to always look the same when I had days where I would feel fat and certainly not consistent. *"If only I had her life, her body, and could even be her, then it would be easy to stay thin"* were the sorts of thoughts I had every time I saw her. It reminded me of a friend in school that used to eat so much packaged food and never gained weight. I was so envious of her at the time and perceived I could never be so lucky.

Well, today I happened to meet this very same mother in person. I was amazed once again by how incorrect my perception can be, and wondered how many other times my assumptions are off target. This mother, while being lovely as a person, has serious food issues! We were talking at a parent-teacher event, at which there was finger food to eat. While I was eating a piece of cake she commented on how lucky I am to be able to eat food "like that" and still stay thin. She, on the other hand, said she had to exercise for two hours a day and just looking at food made her gain weight. I couldn't believe my ears! Was she the same woman I had seen for the last six months and admired and begged to be like? It was another reminder to be careful what I'm envious of. To add to this, the mother in question is also going through a divorce, and came across as very alone and unsupported in life. I felt great compassion for her.

It was a valuable lesson to be happy being myself, rather than wanting to be someone else. I need only ever be envious of myself and the enormous potential I have inside of me. My envy of others, therefore, reveals to me the many untapped jewels within me.

Angel Belief

I'M GLAD TO BE ME.
ME IS ALL I EVER WANT TO BE.
I AM PERFECT JUST AS I AM.

From Elephant to Angel Action

Make a list of all the people you admire or want to be like. Then make a list of what it is you like about them. What qualities and attributes about them do you like? Realize that what you like in others is really what you have within you. We sometimes more easily see the good in others rather than ourselves. These qualities that you admire in others are actually in you right now! Acknowledge this about yourself today.

DAY 56

REST DAY

Today I give thanks for my wonderful arms. I praise my arms for all they carry and for all they do. I admire their shape, their definition, and even the hanging droopy parts. They are beautiful and they are a valued part of me. They are individually mine so I choose to love them.

Extra weight on the arms represents issues in regards to one's mother. I may have many reasons to resent her, but today I think of all the things I appreciate about her. I use the A.N.G.E.L system to release any remnants of resentment and anger and resolve this in myself today.

Today is a day of rest, to acknowledge how much I do for others and how much others do for me. I acknowledge where I mother others, and where others mother me. Today I give gratitude for all that I am and all that I do. I make a list of all the things I have gratitude for. I will use this list on the days when I forget just how lucky I am to be alive.

DAY 57

Elephant Belief

IF I DON'T EAT IT ALL NOW, I WILL MISS OUT.

How many times have I eaten from the point of view that I do not want to miss out? Today I was at my mother-in-law's birthday party and she always serves up the most mouth watering chicken souvlakis I have ever tasted. So I ate, and I ate, and I kept eating until I felt so sick from overeating. My mother-in-law asked me why I was eating so much. I did not take offense, after all I had just downed at least fifteen souvlakis! In complete honesty, I replied, *"Since this is the only night I can eat them, I am eating as many as possible."* She laughed at this and said, *"You do realize you're welcome to take as many as you like home with you, don't you?"* Feeling sillier and fuller than ever, I had to laugh at myself.

It led me to wonder how many times I eat at parties, when I am with others, or even when I am alone so that I can fill the gap inside of me, of all the times I have missed out on things in my life. Perhaps I eat to fill the emptiness of not really getting to know my parents, the gap of not living the life I had always planned, or of never feeling that my life is quite enough. I often feel like I am missing something somewhere. With food, it is so common of us as children to not be allowed to eat our dessert until we finish our food, or we will miss out on dessert altogether! We are taught that if we are not good enough at school, at work, or in relationships, we miss out. Is it any wonder that if some food is before us we dive for it, fearing we will miss out, and thereby lack in our wholeness.

I remind myself there is plenty of food everywhere. I am lucky like this. There is plenty of life everywhere. I am lucky like this. There is plenty of everything I want whenever I want it, and so I will have what I have right now, knowing there is plenty again later should I want more. I get to eat every day, and there is always enough!

Angel Belief

THERE IS AN ABUNDANCE OF FOOD, AND I AM FREE TO HAVE SOME ANY TIME I LIKE WITHOUT FEELING THAT I MISS OUT. I AM ALWAYS SATISFIED.

From Elephant to Angel Action

Write a list of all the things you feel you have missed out on in your life. Be brutally honest with yourself. Write about all the things you are scared of missing out on in the life that lies ahead of you. This is an important exercise to uncover your fears, which may still play out in your eating. As you identify what it is you are actually grieving over having missed or are scared you will miss out on tomorrow, you release the need to project these feelings on to food.

DAY 58

Elephant Belief

I NEED TO PUNISH MYSELF FOR NOT BEING GOOD ENOUGH.

I wonder how many times I punish myself with food, for not feeling I am good enough. I think of all the things about myself I judge around my parenting skills, relationship skills, work practices, and general faults. I am not a perfect human being, only a perfect soul within this life. I have made so many mistakes and still continue to make them. I have broken people's hearts, quit from many things, and lied often in my life. Yes, I am not perfect and I was taught that guilt and shame are positive things to have, because they always keep me "good." What absolute rubbish! How did I believe this for so long?

Feeling constantly that I am not good enough keeps me feeling bad, and when I feel bad I often eat that badness away, covering it up with too much food. Unfortunately even this act is more evidence of how bad I am.

I decide to write a list of all the things I feel I am still not good enough at. It is my secret list and I feel that even though others would try to convince me I am great at these things, I wouldn't believe them. I recognize as I write, so long as I continue to believe I am not good enough, it stops me from gaining all that I really deserve in life. So long as I keep believing I am not a good enough mother, healer, writer, wife, friend, and so many more things, I will continue to sabotage my own happiness and success.

I now choose to set myself free. As I do this, I feel this simple act on this simple day freeing me from at least half of the extra body fat I carry. Skinny people are good enough, and overweight people are good enough too!

Angel Belief

I AM GOOD ENOUGH JUST AS I AM.
I DO MY BEST AND MY EFFORT IS WHAT COUNTS.
I AM WORTHY AND WONDERFUL!

From Elephant to Angel Action

Write down all the things you think you are not good enough at. Make sure you are completely honest with yourself. You either think you ARE good enough at something, or you think you ARE NOT—there is nothing in between. You are choosing in each moment what you think of yourself and your performance in every part of your life. Make a commitment to notice where you are hard on yourself and catch yourself thinking you are not good enough. Noticing is enough to change this. Forgive yourself for not thinking you are good enough and state aloud, *"I forgive myself completely and release this to the universe for correction."*

DAY 59

Elephant Belief

I FEEL UNSUPPORTED IN LIFE.

So many people suffer from back pain. Metaphysically back pain or problems may be associated with feeling unsupported in some way. Most people I suggest this to readily agree and can easily think of someone whose support they feel they need but do not have. I believe through my own reoccurring back issues over certain times in my life, that back pain always reveals that I am not fully supporting myself. It comes back to a universal belief *"I am not enough as I am."* A rejection of some part of myself. In other words, I am harshly judging myself as still not being good enough in my eyes, rather than backing myself.

Supporting myself for how and who I am right now is the doorway to self-acceptance. Supporting myself also includes backing myself even when I react from a limited, conditioned part of myself. It is understanding that I always do the best I can, given my current beliefs. This is the positive statement to keep affirming, *"I love myself, warts and all."* My warts are my limiting beliefs of myself. They are not wrong, however. They just are.

When I judge them as wrong, I am judging myself and letting myself down. When I start supporting myself fully, then I can genuinely start supporting others, and my spine will be strong, self-corrective, flexible, and a perfect transmitter of communication to the rest of my body. When I genuinely begin supporting myself, rather than judging myself, my spine and nervous systems will start supporting the rest of me! This is crucial for my ongoing health and well-being.

Angel Belief

I SUPPORT MYSELF COMPLETELY IN ALL
WAYS AT ALL TIMES.

From Elephant to Angel Action

Today pay attention to all the things you may do that you feel you could have done better. Rather than judging yourself, however, say to yourself, *"I did the best I could in this instance."* So long as you always do your best in every moment, then there is no reason to be negative toward yourself. No matter what mistakes or choices you made today, they were the best you could make today.

Support yourself.

You do not need to tell someone else about your mistakes and have them try to make you feel better. You only need to forgive yourself and acknowledge you always do the best you can do in the here and now.

Back yourself!

In regards to future endeavors, you don't need anyone else to think you are good enough to succeed. You only need think you are worthy and to emotionally support yourself. Make this commitment to yourself right now.

DAY 60

Elephant Belief

WHEN I LOSE WEIGHT, OLD NEGATIVE EMOTIONS ARISE AND I AM AFRAID OF FEELING THEM AGAIN.

I notice as I stay balanced in my thoughts and emotions and truly believe that I can lose weight effortlessly that, in fact, I do! I wrote a list today of new empowering beliefs that will help me to lose those stubborn pounds without needing to eat less or differently. Here are a few:

- My body takes all the goodness from the food I eat, while releasing body fat easily and effortlessly.

- I can eat whatever, whenever I want and be as thin as I like forever.

- There is no connection between the food I eat or the exercise I do with my body and weight.

- I can neutralize everything, anything I want to, any external influences or negative things easily and effortlessly in a moment, so I am no longer affected by them.

- The more I eat, the thinner I become.

However, while I am noticing a marked difference in myself since beginning this process, I am also noticing that as I lose weight I become irritable and grumpy. Negative emotions seem to emerge in me for no particular reason. I am eating well so it cannot be related with my food intake. I am also sleeping well and doing everything else in a kind and gentle manner to myself.

I suddenly remember that when we begin to lose weight (weight that acted as an insulator) old emotions and fears often resurface for clearing. Gaining weight does not clear these things, but rather puts them on hold until we are ready to deal with them. When we lose weight we are often led right back to putting it on again. We fail to realize a potential cause for this is the release of old toxins, both physical and emotional, which our fat was protecting us from in the first place. When we lose weight we need to be prepared for these to be released.

During this time, therefore, I need to nurture myself a little more, slow down in my approach, and most importantly be prepared for this occurrence. I do this by being kind to myself for feeling what I feel and thinking what I think, no matter how negative it may appear. This too shall pass.

I trust that in time my new beliefs will overshadow the past and I will have nothing more to release. For now, I release old things I thought I had dealt with, this time knowing I do not need to avoid them through food. I feel them and they move on and out of me. I recognize as they are released, I become lighter and lighter.

Angel Belief

I EMBRACE MY NEW BELIEFS AROUND FOOD AND WEIGHT AND SUPPORT MYSELF AS I RELEASE OLD UNWANTED EMOTIONS THROUGH LOSING WEIGHT.

From Elephant to Angel Action

Write some incredibly affirming new beliefs today, like I did, to hold you in good stead as you now step into releasing old weight and old fears and emotions attached to this weight. State these new beliefs to yourself for as long as is necessary until you find that you really do believe them. Be free to create any belief you want, without any limiting thoughts such as, *"That cannot possibly be true."* Any belief is possible and with time you will genuinely believe it.

DAY 61

Elephant Belief

BLOCKAGES IN MY ENERGETIC BODY STOP ME FROM RELEASING EXCESS ENERGY SO I GAIN WEIGHT INSTEAD.

From an energetic point of view, all food which I eat is meant to be naturally neutralized by my energy system, and excess food naturally released from my body. What I observe occurring with my medical intuitive x-ray vision is the solar plexus chakra, located just above the navel, naturally transforms the energy of all food into neutral energy. The sacral chakra just below the navel then releases any excess energy that the body does not need to store. After all, the dictionary definition of calories is "units of heat," so it makes sense that the body can easily and effortlessly release excess energy or heat units, because we are not hibernating bears!

Interestingly, I wonder why sometimes the energy system does not do this. Instead it appears to get stuck and excess energy is stored as extra fat rather than being released. The reason is that the solar plexus area is the center of self-esteem and beliefs about self. It is also the center of happiness and joy. Therefore it can be easily affected and thrown off balance, particularly when we are not loving and supporting ourselves, and also when we are not living our life passions. When this chakra is depleted or turned off altogether, then food is not being neutralized effectively, making us more likely to overeat and certainly to gain weight.

The sacral chakra, on the other hand, is the center of relationships, feelings, creativity, sexuality, money beliefs, and decision making. When we have issues in these areas in particular, this center fails to do its job of releasing excess energy. The nervous system then receives an alert signal, informing the fat cells to do their secondary job of keeping us safe. The fat insulates us from the problems of this chakra. Given what this chakra governs and the myriad of problems that people experience in this chakra, is it any wonder everyone is getting fatter?

So, fully understanding this now, I can continue to blame the food because it is easier, but dealing with my deepest self, my emotional self, allows me to transform at a much deeper level. This not only allows me to lose weight but to live with more integrity and harmony.

I KNOW HOW TO KEEP MY ENERGY SYSTEM CORRECTED AND RELEASE ANY EXCESS FOOD THAT I EAT. IT IS AN EASY AND NATURAL PROCESS.

From Elephant to Angel Action

Today, place your left hand on your sacral chakra just below your navel, and your right hand over your solar plexus chakra just above your navel and state the following either in your mind or out loud:

"I release all that I no longer need for my highest good from all directions of time and space. I am the only person able to heal myself. I heal these two areas now and infuse them with healing energy and healing light. My chakras will now do their jobs perfectly to neutralize the energy of food, the energy of emotions, and all other energies, and release that which does not serve me."

Take a deep breath into your sacral chakra and release.

You can do this activity any day when you feel that you need it. Coupled with The Unification Process® described in an earlier chapter, this process will help to make you the master of food, limiting any negative effects and profoundly changing your health.

DAY 62

Elephant Belief

MY BODY IS NOT GOOD ENOUGH AS IT IS AND THIS IS WHY I NEED TO LOSE WEIGHT.

Goals are wonderful when they are based on the positive, such as *"I want to get fit, look great, and feel good more of the time."* On the other hand, if I want this because I feel awful, find myself unbearable, or judge, detest, and dislike where I am right now, what I'm really saying is not the positive statement above. Instead what I am saying is *"I reject who and what I am here and now."* I'm right back to judgment again.

I have noticed something very interesting happens when I reject what is here and now, rejecting the present moment. When I do this I lose any real motivation to change. I become half-hearted about change, and although I might start out motivated, the initial surge dies away leaving me back at my old habits!

Negativity, or moving away from what I do not want, is rarely the breeding ground for the true and genuine momentum I need to grow into something wonderful. Goals are wonderful and powerful when they are based on self-love rather than self-hatred.

The point is to allow the body to do what it does, love it, and trust it. It only slows down because it thinks something is wrong. The only thing that is ever wrong is my attitude and self-perception. So, personally, when it comes to food, I vow to eat healthy, vibrant food because it makes me feel great and alive. That's it, period. No other reasons. I am not going to eat this way to avoid cancer, lose a hundred pounds, or for any other fear-based and judgmental reason. I eat for vitality and joy. When I eat this way, I notice one day just as a cut heals itself without being noticed, that my body finds its natural weight, no matter what I eat.

Angel Belief

I AM WONDERFUL JUST AS I AM; THEREFORE I EAT AND MOVE IN HEALTHY LIFE-GIVING WAYS AS A FORM OF APPRECIATION FOR MYSELF.

From Elephant to Angel Action

Write three new goals today from the perspective that you are already perfect just the way you are. Make them goals which add to your already existing perfection rather than goals to change something you dislike about yourself. Put them up where you can see them for the week. Notice if you are motivated more through the positive intent infused in these goals. Whether you achieve them or not does not matter as you are already whole and complete. Since it does not matter, you will probably achieve them with more ease and grace than you thought possible!

DAY 63

REST DAY

Today is a rest day. Today I give thanks for my chest, for my back, and for my shoulders. They carry so much and nurture others, so today I acknowledge that sometimes I need to be carried and nurtured too.

Extra weight on the upper body represents unresolved issues with my father. I think of all the good things about him today. I use the A.N.G.E.L principle to help change my perspective.

Today I do whatever is required to nurture myself. I spend the day doing the things that I find most nurturing. For me, today, it is going for a relaxing walk, painting, and watching some television when I could be cleaning or doing so many other things. Today is a day for me, guilt free to rejuvenate myself. I go to a special fruit shop out of the way and buy the biggest watermelon I can find that looks deliciously sweet, and I eat the whole thing in one sitting! Yummy! I am so full. When I was a child and I was free to do as I pleased, my nickname was Helen the Watermelon! Today I rest and nurture myself and return to this child-like freedom. I allow the day to be whatever unfolds, and I smile. My shoulders feel lighter, my back less tight, and my chest lifts in joy and fullness.

You can do the same. Do something that nurtures you today.

DAY 64

Elephant Belief

I LACK CONFIDENCE IN MYSELF.

This journey, I now realize, is no different to any other, be it work or relationships. It is a journey of self-confidence and believing in myself.

Yet, can I say I fully believe in my body and consciousness to feel safe, to not gain weight, no matter what? I am still working on it.

In my medical intuitive work I have a belief there is nothing I do not know, no one's health I cannot assess or "read," and I am always right! This may sound like an unfounded belief, but it is mine and it works for me. My self-confidence and self-belief in this area of my life is unshakable, hence I am known for my high accuracy and I am often booked out far in advance. People claim I was born with a gift. I claim we all are born with this intuitive gift. I believe the difference between me and any other person is I believe in myself and *know* I can do it well.

Changing the consciousness of the body is the very same thing. I can eat whatever I want now because I truly have the belief, emotions, and thoughts that are aligned—a knowing.

Confidence is the key, but the challenge is to maintain this confidence no matter what happens around me or within me. Hence, confidence can change and shift from day to day, and in knowing this I keep an eye on it and am aware of it.

In my workshops, I sometimes guide the participants to do an exercise I was shown by one of the Qi Gong masters with whom I trained. The process involves using the mind to grow one hand longer than the other. I first demonstrate and people are always astounded that I have actually managed to achieve it. Then everyone else tries and they too are amazed that they can also do it. People think it must be a trick, but really it is a demonstration of confidence. The Qi Gong master who taught this to me told me I would become a better healer from doing this technique every day rather than practicing healing on others. He impressed upon me that it was more important than anything else I could do, in order to be a good practitioner. This practice has indeed given me high confidence in all areas of my life. After all, if I can physically grow my own hand with my mind, what else am I capable of achieving? According to him confidence is the key and over the years I have discovered he is right.

Angel Belief

I HAVE CONFIDENCE IN MYSELF AND KNOW I CAN DO ANYTHING I FEEL CONFIDENT TO DO AND BE IN MY LIFE.

From Elephant to Angel Action

Anyone can do the technique of growing their hand to see how much confidence they have or lack. The more your hand grows the more confidence you have.

Here's how you do it:

Put your two hands together, palm pressing upon palm. Close your eyes and ask one of your hands to grow. You can say, *"I ask this hand to grow. It is growing now. It is growing longer and longer."* You ask and think it to grow for about five minutes and then check to see if it has. Imagine in your mind it is growing. Feel it growing longer and longer.

Did you manage to make it grow? Do not worry if you did, it will go back to normal eventually. If you did not yet make it grow, keep trying. Remember this is a test of your confidence levels. Keep practicing!

CONGRATULATIONS!

**You are almost at the end of your eighty-one day journey.
For the next two weeks you will more deeply explore the twelve power
centres of the body. They were explained in Day 27.**

Working with and energizing these twelve centers will help substantially
with shifting the consciousness of the body. These twelve power centers are
tremendous at removing many old beliefs. All human problems are related to one
of these twelve areas. These twelve sacred healing centers of the body are located
at dominant nerve centers within the body, as described by Catherine Ponder in
her book, *The Healing Secrets of the Ages*. I developed a meditation to balance these
twelve important centers in the body a few years ago when I completely lost
my voice and was told the only way to get it back was through surgery to have
a giant nodule removed. After listening to this meditation every day, within two
weeks my voice was fully restored! I was so impressed I recorded this meditation
for others. It is called *HORMONE HARMONY: A daily meditation to heal your
hormones and reenergize your life*. So many people write to me, telling me of the
radical improvement to their health as a result of listening to this meditation track
daily. I felt it a crucial thing to explore these twelve sacred healing centers as a part
of my eighty-one days of self-reflection.

You will then complete your eighty-one days with the four levels of consciousness—victim, metaphysical, mystical, and master. Your journey of eighty-one
days will then officially be complete.

DAY 65

Elephant Belief

I DO NOT TRUST MYSELF AND ALL THAT I HAVE TO OFFER TO THE WORLD. I ASK MYSELF, IS IT ENOUGH? AM I ENOUGH? I DOUBT MYSELF.

Today I am contemplating the important role of **FAITH**. Even given how far I have come, I find myself thinking perhaps it is easier to just go back to dieting and listening to the experts rather than believing I am a powerful creator in my own life.

As I woke up this morning, I felt in turmoil. Having been writing this book for so long and almost being done, I found myself thinking, *"Do I publish this controversial book or is it too much for people? Why can't I have written a self-help book that just gives people another prescription for weight loss?"* It all seemed too hard.

Later in the morning, while in my exercise class, I incorrectly stepped off the aerobic stepper and seriously sprained my right ankle, tearing some ligaments. I know that my right ankle represents stepping into my future and allowing myself to step forward into a new beginning in my life. Here I am writing a book about trusting your inner self and body to do what is required of it, yet do I really have FAITH in this approach? It is one thing to preach to others and quite another thing to believe and practice my own approach.

Having injured myself, my first thought was, *"I am going to get fat. I can't exercise. I'm going to sit around all day and get fat!"* What a test of faith. It was also a timely reminder that I need to have faith in my ability to stand up tall in front of others and present a different approach to eating while supporting myself rather than seeking approval from others.

It can feel so overwhelming to begin to trust and have faith in a new approach such as the one this book offers, when I have been conditioned my whole life to believe that excess food turns into fat. Today is the day I begin to truly have faith in this way of being. I have listened to the message of my foot, and I will no longer avoid the path I was placed here to walk. I will walk it, and have faith in a higher power to guide me. I can think I have made the shift, but if there is even a seed of doubt something will come right in and show me otherwise. Without my foot injury perhaps I would never have recognized this doubt in myself and it would have caused more trouble further down the track. In my awareness of it, I now make the decision to do away with doubt and embrace the full ability that FAITH has to offer me.

Angel Belief

I HAVE NO DOUBT IN THIS METHOD AND NO DOUBT IN MYSELF. I RELEASE IT ALL NOW AND EMBRACE ONLY FAITH IN MYSELF AND THIS APPROACH AS BEING RIGHT FOR ME.

From Elephant to Angel Action

The mind power of **FAITH** is located in the center of the brain at the pineal gland. Imagine this area in your brain glowing brightly. Imagine energizing the faith center in your brain with vibrant healing and balancing light. Keep focusing the light in this region until it feels full, vibrant, and healthy.

Affirm: *"Divine faith expresses itself fully through me now. I have faith in myself, in the Divine, and in my body. It is done now!"*

DAY 66

Elephant Belief

I LACK THE STRENGTH TO ACHIEVE ALL THAT I DESIRE AND TO BE THE BEST THAT I CAN BE.

Today, I was at martial art training, and we were required to perform spinning kicks low to the ground. This is incredibly difficult, and even the black belts can struggle as it requires spinning very quickly landing on your palms, then finishing the kick and standing up again, all done at lightning speed. I think because I have been journaling my experience in this book, that instead of panicking as I may have normally done, I focused in on what I wanted to achieve.

I then proceeded to use a technique that I teach at my workshops whereby I can access other people's formula for success. If someone is great at something I want to be great at, I just need to access the mastery in them, in order to also be as good as they are. Essentially the technique involves stepping into someone else's Morphic Field and accessing their energetic blueprint.

It may sound strange, but this is how it worked at martial arts that day: I imagined in my mind that I was stepping into the energy and expertise of the head instructor. I kept chanting to myself that I would do it just like him. When it was my turn, people were astonished at my speed, precision, and agility. I had performed my kick like a professional! Everyone obviously assumed it was just luck, so when it was my turn again, I again imagined I was the head instructor and told myself I would do it just the way he did it. I did a perfect kick again, and again, and again. I was just as amazed with myself as the others were amazed with me. It proved to me that inner strength and mastery can be created through thought just like anything else, and need not be something I slave away at achieving. It is mine, here and now, if I am ready and willing to use my thoughts to create it.

Angel Belief

TO ME, STRENGTH IS ALL ABOUT HEALTH, VITALITY, PERSISTENCE, SUCCESS AND A COMPLETE BELIEF IN ONLY THE GOOD.

From Elephant to Angel Action

The mind power of **STRENGTH** is located between the adrenal glands in the small of the back. Imagine this area in your back glowing brightly. Imagine energizing the strength center in your body with vibrant healing and balancing light. Keep focusing the light in this region until it feels full, vibrant, and healthy.

Affirm: *"Divine strength expresses itself fully through me now. I have strength in myself, in the Divine, and in my body. It is done now!"*

DAY 67

Elephant Belief

I NEED JUDGMENT TO MOTIVATE ME FORWARD.

I was watching a television show last night based on contestants competing for who can lose the most weight. I watched as their fitness trainer made constant statements of condemnation toward them and expressed great disappointment in their recent eating behavior. His judgment of them was that they were weak and undisciplined. He dished out a thick layer of guilt and the women on the show felt it.

Guilt and judgment can be one way to motivate oneself, but it certainly does not work for me. I need to feel great in order to get the most out of myself. Likewise, at the gym, I hear women all the time saying they are exercising because of what they ate yesterday. I hear so often parents around me expressing negativity and judgment to their children about what they are eating.

Judgment, located in the stomach area of the body, can greatly affect digestion. Is it any wonder so many people these days suffer from digestive problems? People take all sorts of supplements and other remedies to try correcting these conditions, but it all begins with peace and acceptance. We need to stop judging ourselves. After all it is basic psychology that positive reinforcement always works best, rather than negative reinforcement.

I have not once had an overweight client step into my consultation room that did not feel intense judgment toward themselves for being overweight. The labels they carry for themselves and others who are overweight could fill a scrapbook. Until they erase these labels, they will not find themselves or the solution they seek to their weight loss. Weight loss needs to be made of forgiveness, not self-condemnation.

Angel Belief

I RELEASE ALL JUDGMENT AND EMBRACE LOVE AND FORGIVENESS FOR MYSELF AROUND FOOD.

From Elephant to Angel Action

The mind power of **JUDGMENT** is located in the stomach in the solar plexus near the pancreas. Imagine this area in your body glowing brightly. Imagine energizing the judgment center in your body with vibrant healing and balancing light. Keep focusing light in this region until it feels full, vibrant, and healthy.

Affirm: *"Divine judgment expresses itself fully through me now. I have the discernment to know what is best for the divine me, and for my body. It is done now!"*

DAY 68

LOVE IS SOMETHING I NEED TO EARN FROM OTHERS. LOVE IS CONDITIONAL.

Having a high self-esteem means I love and appreciate myself as I am today. This means I fully accept myself and my body. Accepting myself does not mean I will never have goals of self-improvement. In fact the very opposite is true. When I love and accept myself I can more easily do what is required to improve my body and my life. It is very possible to have a high self-esteem and look in the mirror and state I look and feel fat. The difference between having a high self-esteem and saying this and a low self-esteem and saying this is high self-esteem has no attachment to the outcome. A person with a high self-esteem does not need to be slimmer in order to accept themselves, whereas someone with a low self-esteem, needs to look good to feel good.

I also learn today that I sometimes see giving of love as all or nothing—either I look after and love everyone else to my own detriment, or I am selfish and put myself before others. I do not really believe this, however. I don't really believe that I need to be selfish in order to look after myself, versus giving all my love away to others. I do, on the other hand, believe that whatever I give, I also receive. So when I give my time and love to others with no strings attached and expect nothing in return, I receive more love in return. Likewise when I give lots of love to myself I am full.

I find that when I have compassion for overweight people, I also allow a compassion and love for myself. It is like I am saying to myself, *"If you were ever to become that overweight, I will still love you."* Change grows best and fastest in the fertile ground of love. Love is all there is, and unconditional love is not something I need to look for in the world, but something I can be a leader in. It is something I give to myself and then to others.

Angel Belief

I KEEP MY LOVE BANK FULL AND PLENTIFUL KNOWING THERE IS ABUNDANT LOVE FOR ALL. THROUGH LOVE, ALL THINGS ARE POSSIBLE.

From Elephant to Angel Action

The mind power of **LOVE** is located in the chest, near the thymus gland. Imagine this area in your body glowing brightly. Imagine energizing the love center in your body with vibrant healing and balancing light. Keep focusing the light in this region until it feels full, vibrant, and healthy.

Affirm: *"Divine love expresses itself fully through me now. I have complete unconditional love for myself, for the Divine in me, and for my body. It is done now!"*

DAY 69

I CAN SPEAK SO NEGATIVELY
TO MYSELF AND OTHERS.

The words I speak have great power. If I speak negative words, I create negative outcomes. I am reminded today to always praise myself and others, and to look for the good, even in the seemingly bad.

This morning I blew up at my son for some small insignificant reason. As I got in the car with him, still fuming, I suddenly realized I was not really angry at him, but angry with myself for a mistake I had made earlier that day. I explained this to him and then said, *"Wasn't it wonderful that this just happened?"* Confused he asked why this would be a good thing. It was a good thing I replied, *"Because it helped me to learn more about myself and, every time I learn about my behaviors, I improve."* I could tell my answer made him think, and it made us both smile. I could just as easily have spent the rest of the day in penance for this earlier act. Instead, my words of praise spoken about myself changed the whole situation.

How often do you overeat for the wrong reasons and then spend the rest of the day eating more just to hurt yourself, as well as speaking words of negativity about your behavior? How often do you speak with friends about someone you know who has gained weight? We are, seemingly, always ready to speak the negative about ourselves and others. Our gossip of famous people and their weight is another example of this.

At one point in my life I had gained some extra weight. A doctor I was seeing at the time commented how fantastic this was as it was exactly what my nervous system needed in order to heal. I had never thought of it from this perspective, but sure enough my healing was quick and smooth, and after I was well I lost that extra weight effortlessly.

You never know what is really occurring at a cellular level in your body, so you need to trust, and you do this through your spoken words. Your words have power and as this power is executed, your life expands. When you speak the truth and speak the positive, you empower yourself and your body.

Angel Belief

**I SPEAK ONLY WORDS OF PRAISE AND LIGHT,
KNOWING MY WORDS HAVE POWER.
WORDS OF FORGIVENESS HELP TO HEAL
ANY NEGATIVE WORDS I SPEAK.**

From Elephant to Angel Action

The mind faculty of **POWER** is located at the base of the tongue in the throat near the thyroid gland. Imagine this area in your throat glowing brightly. Imagine energizing this power center in your body with vibrant healing and balancing light. Keep focusing the light in this region until it feels full, vibrant, and healthy.

Affirm: *"Divine power expresses itself fully through me now. I access the deep inner power within myself, within the Divine, and within my body. It is done now!"*

DAY 70

REST DAY

Today is a rest day. I remind myself that I can have a rest day whenever I want to. I remind myself today to always give myself rest days. Rest days are important days to renew and give thanks and praise. They are days to consciously slow down and say to myself *"Well done!"*

Today I give praise to my throat. It says so much, and yet sometimes expresses so little. Today is my day to express all that I feel and to know that the universe hears me, even if no one else does. And I hear me too!

Together let's give gratitude for the gift of self-expression. How lucky we are to be able to speak and communicate in so many ways.

DAY 71

Elephant Belief

IMAGINING A NEW ME IS NOT ENOUGH TO MAKE IT HAPPEN.

Imagination is an alive essence. I do not need to force things to happen through it, like imagining something to be and trying to make it happen. Instead I am reminded that I ask through my imagination center what needs to happen for healing, balance and inner peace to occur and it answers me. If I wake up feeling tired or unwell, I do not imagine myself better, but I ask for inner guidance on what will return me to balance, and I am always provided with the correct answer for me.

Imagination is not a pretend, forced mind power. Instead it is an alive and guiding one. Imagination provides the vehicle for the secret language of the mind, body, and soul. The brain sends us messages through images, often metaphorical ones. Its language is not one of words, but of pictures. This is the reason we dream such unusual things. They are not imaginary, as in make-believe, but alive as a valid form of communication.

The more I listen to my imagination, the more I expand my understanding of self, my life, and the best way forward into the future. When I listen to and follow the path of my imagination mind power, apart from generating healing of every kind, I avoid the need for my body to communicate to me through illness. The more I listen to the messages of my imagination, the less I need to listen to my body as my wake-up call.

When I help facilitate people to heal, I receive images and metaphors in my imagination that relate back to the client's issues and problems. It is through my imagination that I appear psychic and to know things about people without being told anything about them. I then use this information to gain the appropriate guidance for their higher healing. This is why the healing is often successful. I am receiving the best approach through my imagination, rather than using my logic to force a healing. Instead of forcefully willing people to heal, I allow their incredible intelligence to guide me through my imagination to their place of wellness. Now, this is all happening in my own mind, so when I first began working this way, I very much doubted that it was really producing results in people. How could it? However, every single person I have ever treated, either through a telephone consultation or in person, has at the very least reported feeling lighter, calmer, and more peaceful after a medical intuitive healing session. Healing results astound both my clients and myself, as all sorts of disorders that could not be treated any other way often vanish. When I explored further how this unusual method of healing works, I found it was because I was not using my imagination to merely imagine a healing taking place. My imagination was the medium through which the body and consciousness of each client was communicating to me what it required to be well again.

When I train my medical intuitive students, although I teach them a great deal about the body and energy system, I always remind them that when they enter into a healing relationship with a client, they almost need to forget all they have learned and allow their imagination to speak to them what the client needs. Failing to do this, it is very easy for a trained practitioner to easily project onto clients what is wrong with them.

In relationship to my body today, I will ask my imagination center to let me know through quiet moments of contemplation what is required in order for me to change to this new way of being so that I may eat anything with no negative consequences. I must believe that receiving an answer is possible either through my visual senses, my sense of knowing, hearing, or feeling. I will trust it to be true. This information is all the information I need to know. I will follow its guidance—my inner guidance. It never lets me down.

Angel Belief

I LISTEN TO AND FOLLOW THE GUIDANCE
OF MY IMAGINATION. IT IS ALIVE AND WISE
AND OFFERS ME THE ANSWERS I NEED TO
EVERY QUESTION.

From Elephant to Angel Action

The mind power of **IMAGINATION** is located between the eyes, near the pituitary gland. Imagine this area in your body glowing brightly. Imagine energizing the imagination center in your body with vibrant healing and balancing light. Keep focusing the light in this region until it feels full, vibrant, and healthy.

Affirm: *"Divine imagination expresses itself fully through me now. I have the most amazing imagination that flows constantly through me, is connected to the Divine, and infuses my body in every way. It is done now!"*

DAY 72

Elephant Belief

I'LL NEVER BE FREE TO BE ME.

I am relieved to have traveled this far on my journey and truly believe I am free to be me. I am free to eat as I please and what I please. I feel free to finally understand that doing this does not mean I will become fat and ugly, but it means I will simply be me. I feel free to finally have this understanding, and I trust my deep mind power of understanding to now guide me forward at all times. It will reveal to me what is best for me to eat at any given moment. Food is plentiful, and I know that I will always be looked after, always be safe in the world, and always find the tools that I require to be well, whole, and complete.

I believe and know on every level of my being that divine understanding truly does reside inside me, and it will always, and I mean *always*, talk to me and through me. I can never make a mistake again, because every decision I make brings me to new understanding of my true nature and my true self. I now understand that my body needs my love and support, not my anger and resentment. I now understand that the people around me, who cannot understand me or this approach, need love and compassion, not anger and judgment. I finally UNDERSTAND!

Divine understanding is a powerful mind power. It is the power often called the Third Eye, or psychic power. But it is not so mysterious or new age. Rather the power of understanding is directly related to inner knowing and intuitive hunches.

Angel Belief

I AM FREE TO BE ME.
I UNDERSTAND THIS AND MY INTUITIVE
UNDERSTANDING NOW LEADS THE WAY TO A
NEW LIFE AND A NEW WAY OF BEING.

From Elephant to Angel Action

The mind power of **UNDERSTANDING** is located in the front brain, just above the eyes. Imagine this area in your brain glowing brightly. Imagine energizing the understanding center in your body with vibrant healing and balancing light. Keep focusing the light in this region until it feels full, vibrant, and healthy.

Affirm: *"Divine understanding expresses itself fully through me now. I have complete understanding through my intuition and I listen to it in every way, and I listen to my body's deep understanding about what it wants to eat. It is done now!"*

DAY 73

I WILL GET THE BODY I WANT
THROUGH WILLPOWER.

We all want so much. I know I do. I think I am fairly ambitious and driven, and yet as I have grown older, I observe how this attitude has not always served me well. Sometimes, to the point of obsession, I have focused on creating the next thing and achieving the next outcome. Many people might think this is great, but within me no matter what I have achieved, it still feels as if it is never enough. When I overcome huge obstacles and get what I think I want, I find I only look for something else to want. Such is the mind power of will. Will is a wonderful force when used with kind self-understanding and a clear direction, but left to its own devices, it often causes much conflict both in the mind and the body.

Most weight-loss techniques or approaches on the market today are based on willful approaches. You will your body, you make it do what you want it to do, because you have suddenly decided it is what you want: to be thin. You have decided (not usually based on your internal wisdom) that you must lose weight at all costs, and you will do whatever you decide is required to make it happen.

At the end of the day, all of our many wants reveal something deeper about our heart's longings and about the things we truly want, yet believe we cannot have. All we ever really want is love, acceptance, and to feel a part of the whole. So long as this eludes us we look for it in the external world.

A friend recently asked me whether I felt loved by my parents as I was growing up. I thought about this for a minute and my own answer surprised me. I did feel loved by them in terms of my inner worth and personality, but I never felt good enough for them in regards to how I looked. It explained to me why no matter how much I validated the internal me, and felt worthy, lovable, and complete on the inside, I still chased the outside perfect look. It was still of vital importance for me to hold on to my external appearance, no matter what. This really helped me to understand why my willpower was so strong. Surprisingly other people viewed this willful approach in me as wonderful and reinforced it in me further.

Now I know better. I know that divine will when it acts without divine understanding has once, and can again if I allow it, get me into an obsession-like space from which I do not feel free to return. I understand that without the cues of my inner wise woman, my outer persona will always be looking for the next best external promise made by a world and industry that is focused on results at any cost, and outer perfection as its motivator. My health is the most important thing to me these days, because being strong and healthy means I can do the things I really came to do here on Earth—namely, play and have fun! Will can be very useful, however, when it is led first by deep and honest understanding. Willpower then helps me to take the action I am shown is good for me.

Angel Belief

AS I ALLOW A DEEPER UNDERSTANDING TO LEAD IN MY LIFE, MY WILL LEADS ME TO TAKE ACTION.

From Elephant to Angel Action

The mind power of **WILL** is located in the center of the front brain. Imagine this area in your brain glowing brightly. Imagine energizing the will center in your body with vibrant healing and balancing light. Keep focusing the light in this region until it feels full, vibrant, and healthy.

Affirm: *"Divine will expresses itself fully through me now. I harness the power of my will to guide me in my life, and know it is completely one with divine will, and expresses itself through my body at all times. It is done now!"*

DAY 74

BECAUSE I CAN EAT ANYTHING I WANT AND NOT GAIN WEIGHT, I WILL EAT LOTS OF PROCESSED FOOD ALL THE TIME—WHY NOT, SINCE I CAN?

While my whole approach throughout this book is to eat anything I want, today I had another insight that went one step further than this again. Yes, while I can eat anything I like and not gain weight, I now understand that this is a place to journey through, but certainly not the destination.

First, I needed to believe that to love myself meant no longer punishing myself, depriving myself, or giving myself guilt trips over food. Having achieved this, I spent almost two whole years eating anything and everything that I possibly wanted. I probably ate the food I had not allowed myself to eat all the years prior. In this process I did not gain any weight. In fact I seemed to stay the same weight no matter what I ate. I believed I had found the end of the rainbow.

Today I suddenly understand that true self-love is not just about being able to eat anything I want, but rather about giving myself what I really want in life. When I do this, food just falls off the radar of importance. It becomes something I do, not something I am. Divine order is about knowing what your appetites are really stating. Order in mind and body allows the false cravings to fall away, and allows me to desire the purest food. Now I know that, when I love myself, I commit to eating more life-giving foods, helping my body with good quality fuel. This is easy to do because my thoughts, emotions, and life are on track.

Can I eat anything I like and not gain weight? Sure. Do I always have to eat rubbish in this case? No. Because I love my body, love myself, and love life.

Angel Belief

I KNOW I CAN EAT ANYTHING I LIKE, AND BEING FREE TO DO THIS, I NOW WILLINGLY CHOOSE TO EAT MORE NATURAL FOOD MOST OF THE TIME.

From Elephant to Angel Action

The mind power of **ORDER** is located at a large nerve center just behind the navel. Imagine this area in your stomach glowing brightly. Imagine energizing the order center in your body with vibrant healing and balancing light. Keep focusing the light in this region until it feels full, vibrant, and healthy.

Affirm: *"Divine order expresses itself fully through me now. I have complete order in my life, in my body, and in eating. It is done now!"*

DAY 75

I AM ALWAYS SEARCHING FOR THE BEST APPROACH TO EATING AND WHEN I NEVER FIND IT, I LOSE ENTHUSIASM FOR CHANGE.

I find, without enthusiasm to infuse my every moment, I am only half committed to anything I do, and eventually my self-discipline to continue wanes. With this, my results also never appear. Whenever I have started a new diet or eating approach, I am so enthusiastic. I believe it is "the one." I believe that it is finally the approach that will save me, make my life easy, and I will finally commit to it for life and not have to worry about my weight ever again. So I begin, and with this beginning I get results, but after a few weeks, I start to lose my enthusiasm. I begin to see that what seemed initially like the best approach in the world was just a desperate me looking to be saved again. I see myself as a problem to be solved, and each and every time it seems something will "solve" me, I jump for it convinced *this is finally it*. But it never is. I know that I will eventually become bored and give up. Each time losing faith and trust in myself, and each time sinking a little bit lower as I return back to searching. Always searching.

I have come to understand that divine zeal, or enthusiasm, is not something I must create, but instead something I must listen to as a sign. It is a sign post to what I am truly meant for compared with what is a fake longing in me. If my enthusiasm fades away, I know it was just me looking in the wrong place again. True zeal is to have life and vigor, excitement and deep gratitude for where I find myself in life. It is eating with gusto and love, rather than longing and emptiness. True zeal and enthusiasm is being in the right place at the right time, tapping into the synchronicity of the universe, and allowing myself to go forward in life, easily and effortlessly. And it stays when I am doing the right thing for me.

When I eat now, knowing how and what I eat has nothing to do with my body and everything to do with my soul, I eat what feeds my enthusiasm and zeal. If I am so enthusiastic about eating, it will nourish and support me, and never remain on me as extra fat. If on the other hand I only eat for relaxation, boredom, and just because food is available, there is no life energy in this food. In this knowledge I abandon finding the best expert approach and just eat with joy.

Angel Belief

I ALLOW MY ENTHUSIASM TO GUIDE ME TO THE BEST FOOD CHOICES AND TO MY BEST LIFE.

From Elephant to Angel Action

The mind power of **ZEAL** is located at the base of the brain in the back of the neck at the medulla. Imagine this area in your brain glowing brightly. Imagine energizing the zeal center in your brain with vibrant healing and balancing light. Keep focusing the light in this region until it feels full, vibrant, and healthy.

Affirm: *"Divine zeal expresses itself fully through me now. I have zeal for life. I have enthusiasm for my life and I enthusiastically look after myself. It is done now!"*

DAY 76

Elephant Belief

I CANNOT SURRENDER MY WEIGHT TO A HIGHER POWER. I DON'T FULLY TRUST YET.

I know I can fight and struggle to create the body I want, but today I want to learn to surrender instead. Today I give my body the clear and simple intent that I am now at a point in my development and self-creation where I am ready to begin losing weight. I do not **will** it to happen. I listen to my **understanding** of what this will require. I have **faith** that it will happen. I have **enthusiasm** in the process. Now, all I need to do is **LET GO**. Once the intent is created all I ever need to do is let it go.

I feel I need to dig even deeper. Rather than just give the directive around weight loss, I need to be clear about what it is I am really wanting through being thinner than I am now. With all the clearing I have been doing through my journaling, I am now very clear that what I really want is the vitality and energy to feel great in my body, to just eat when I eat, and to love and feel free to move as I please. I want to feel alive and free. So I let all this go, too. The minute I want something, I really need to remember that through my mere wanting I already set something into motion. It is already in existence in Divine Mind. I hold onto things only when I think I cannot have them.

No one wants me to be overweight. No one wants me to be unhappy. I deserve to have what I want, and through letting go and surrendering what I think I want most, I am set free. If it is truly meant for me, it will be delivered. It will arrive.

One day, not so long ago, I decided I wanted to go back to college and become an osteopath. I decided I wanted it, and I wanted it now! I was obsessed by it. I kept looking it up on the internet, and thinking about it incessantly. Then one day I was lying down meditating and I asked, *"Is this what God wants for me on Earth?"* I thought I heard a no, but this was not good enough. I had decided I wanted it! Goodness knows why, but I did. It took a few weeks of inner struggle to understand, if I really did want it, and it was best for me, by letting it go it would come back to me. I thought I had to keep it close to me and make it happen. So I let it go. Am I meant to become an osteopath right now? No, but I could only really discover this through letting go of my need and my obsession with it. Sometimes what I think I want is just there to distract me or show me a deeper longing. Through the act of surrender, what is truly mine always comes back.

Angel Belief

THROUGH SURRENDER, I GET WHAT IS MEANT TO BE MINE. I SURRENDER MY WEIGHT AND ANY REMAINING FOOD ISSUES, TRUSTING THEM TO BE HEALED.

From Elephant to Angel Action

The mind power of **ELIMINATION** is located in the organs of elimination in the lower back. Imagine this area in your back glowing brightly. Imagine energizing the elimination center in your body with vibrant healing and balancing light. Keep focusing light in this region until it feels full, vibrant, and healthy.

Affirm: *"Divine elimination expresses itself fully through me now. I have the ability to let go of all that I no longer need in my body, in my eating habits, and in my life. Elimination is the order of the day. It is done now!"*

DAY 77

REST DAY

Today I praise my head and my face. I revel in the wonder of my senses—sight, hearing, taste, touch, and smell. I affirm how lucky I am to know what I know and to be who I am. Today I focus on increasing the joy of my senses. I pay attention a little more to all that I taste, without getting as distracted by sounds and sights around me. I close my eyes today as I eat and really taste the food. I imagine being an alien who has just tasted food for the first time. How lucky am I?

I am so grateful for my sense of taste. I look at the food I eat today as if looking at it for the first time ever. I wonder if I really were an alien and all foods were equal, what food would I choose to eat? Would I choose white food or colorful food? I wonder. I give thanks that I am not an alien! Instead I am wonderfully human. I give thanks for my wondrous brain that gives me free will and knowledge, and does the best it can. I give myself permission to love myself, to love food, and to love my life.

DAY 78

Elephant Belief

I REACT TO CERTAIN FOODS.
I CRAVE CERTAIN FOODS.

I am fascinated by the increase in eating intolerances that exist among people in this day and age. It seems to have blown out of proportion. From gluten free to dairy free, everybody seems to have some food that their body appears not to cope with anymore. But what if the very food we are avoiding is a message of something much deeper we are missing in our lives? I asked my inner wisdom this question today and received a list of foods and their metaphysical meanings. Whether it is accurate or not according to the experts does not interest me, but what does is that it seems to me logical that all these intolerances are not simply due to a change in the environment, but rather a change in thinking.

At a recent get-together with friends, I was mortified when one of the children stated they could never eat wheat again and asked the rest of the children what food they were not allowed to ever eat again. They all had at least one food they mentioned! What beliefs we are planting in them at this age, and how this will impact on them as adults, I do not know. My theory is to allow foods your body no longer wants to leave of their own accord through love rather than through force. If the body does not like wheat anymore, it will naturally steer away from it, when more nutritional or appropriate foods are available instead. Gentle change through love is always going to inspire life rather than change based on fear and consequence.

Here is my very brief list of foods and what an intolerance to them may represent on a deeper level. This is purely my interpretation, and I offer it only as a guide to deeper self-understanding. The list can also be useful for understanding cravings, not only intolerances.

Wheat: What do I lack faith in at the moment? Myself perhaps, and how to best move forward in life? I choose instead to have faith in myself and the higher power that illuminates me.

Dairy: Do I feel connected to Mother Earth and to this life, or am I wanting to go back to spirit form where it all seems so much easier? I understand, instead, that I belong here and find my love and connection once more to this life and to Earth.

Sugar: Am I living my life from the place of pure joy and fun or am I too serious about life? I have come here to play and have fun. Joy is the reason I am here, not to save the world. The only person that needs saving is myself, through just having fun.

Fruit: When I wake up in the morning do I feel alive and excited about the day ahead, or am I always looking for some future moment to make my life happy? All I really need is in the here and now. All I need is in this moment. I focus on it and my aliveness for life returns.

Meat: Am I taking enough time to truly nurture myself through the act of doing nothing, or do I constantly push myself to achieve the next thing, and then the next? I remind myself to be comfortable with doing nothing and allow self-nurturing to be a natural and necessary part of my life.

Egg: Am I birthing and creating what I have truly come to do in this life, or am I procrastinating and looking for my self-worth in all the wrong places? I dig a little deeper to find the area in my life where my true creative talents can be put to best use. I begin to allow creativity to flow from within me again.

Fish: Am I impatient with waiting for either inner guidance or life to show me where I belong? I know what I do not want, but am still unsure as to what I do want, and certainly won't wait long enough to find out. So I keep filling the empty space with my own fantasies. I decide today that it is worth waiting for the right answer to come to me, all in good time. Meanwhile, while I am waiting, I will have some fun, put my feet up, and be patient.

Chocolate: Whose love do I crave? Which relationship feels like it has lost its luster and its deeper appeal? Perhaps I am looking at my current partner, or lack thereof. But instead I am looking at myself in the mirror. It is the person looking back at me in the mirror that I need to reconnect to. I need to get to know myself on a deeper level.

Crunchy food: Do I need to fight and strive to always get what I want? Do I need to keep up with the crowd? I don't really. I am a unique individual and what I desire will come to me if I simply let go.

Fried food: Does my life feel too hard and too full of activities? Does it feel as though I never have time off from the responsibilities of life? It is time to make space for me. It is time to stop playing the victim about how I never have enough time and to create time. Time is in my control. I can choose what I do with it. I choose to spend my time more wisely.

Cakes and pastries: What am I protecting myself from? Am I afraid to love and be loved in order to protect myself from loss? Yes, all things, including bodies, are impermanent, but I am here now and those whom I love are here now too, whether in a body or not. We are always safe and immortal.

Soy: Why do I search for superficial happiness when true and genuine happiness is here and waiting for me to embrace? I am still seeking external worth and to fit into the culture of the day. As I now let this go, I instead honor all that is within me waiting to be revealed. I honor the masculine and feminine qualities equally and life becomes easier and more joyful. Life can be fulfilling in an easy and straightforward way when I allow it to be.

Angel Belief

MY FOOD INTOLERANCES OR CRAVINGS REVEAL SOMETHING DEEPER ABOUT MY THINKING AND MY LIFE. AS I EMBRACE EACH INSIGHT I BECOME FREE TO EAT WHATEVER I LIKE.

From Elephant to Angel Action

The mind power of **LIFE** is located in the generative organs. Imagine this area in your body glowing brightly. Imagine energizing the life center in your body with vibrant healing and balancing light. Keep focusing the light in this region until it feels full, vibrant, and healthy.

Affirm: *"Divine life expresses itself fully through me now. I harness the fullness of my life and live according to my inner desires. I can have everything I desire in life. It is mine now! It is done now!"*

DAY 79

Elephant Belief

I AM A VICTIM WHEN IT COMES TO FOOD AND EATING.

I have read many times about the four levels of consciousness and do my best to live from the higher levels as much as possible. Today I am reminded of them in relation to food. If they apply to other areas of life, then logically they can be just as relevant with food. What are they? They are as follows:

1. Victim

Life happens **to me**, and I am powerless. At this level there is someone outside of myself that I can blame.

2. Metaphysical

I begin to understand that life happens **as me**. I am powerful and direct what occurs in my life through my thoughts and actions. I can think certain things and use forces outside of the physical to direct my life. At this level I have both control and responsibility over my life.

3. Mystical

There is a greater power than I and it works **through me** to create all that I am. This power is only good. Yet at this stage this greater power is still outside of me and separate to me.

4. Master

Life and I are one and the same. We are united. At this stage, the Divine is me, **as me**. The Divine and I are one and the same. No separation exists, only oneness and wholeness.

Today I will explore any remnants of the victim attitude within me in relation to food. I must admit I do sometimes whine about why this process has to be so hard and long winded, when technically we were all born knowing this information already. Why can't I have kept and known the wisdom of my body to cope with ANYTHING I put in it, from birth right up until now? After all it was Jesus who taught his disciples, nothing external can affect you, only your internal reaction and perception to things can. His wisdom applied to food means that food as an external thing has no inherent power of its own. Its only power is that given to it through thought.

As a victim to food, it is easy to believe that food has all the power and I am powerless against it. If I eat something bad, I will gain weight. It has nothing to do with my thinking; it is just the way it is. However, this is neither a responsible nor empowered way to live my life around food. There is NOTHING in the universe that has more power than the power I have to change and shift everything through my thoughts. Today having come so far in this journey, I will release any remaining victim energy and victim thoughts that disempower me around food. I am free to choose what food becomes for me and so it is.

Angel Belief

**FOOD HAS NO INHERENT POWER OF ITS OWN.
I DECIDE WHAT FOOD WILL MEAN TO ME
AND DO FOR ME.**

From Elephant to Angel Action

Write any victim perceptions that are still lurking within you in relation to food. For example, include a description of any body parts that you dislike but feel powerless to change, any lingering beliefs about your inability to eat anything you like and lose weight, and any foods you still fear eating. These are all based on your perceptions based on cultural norms. They are not the truth. Next to each thing on your list write, *"This is not the truth. The truth is I have the power to choose."*

DAY 80

Elephant Belief

I AM NOT POWERFUL ENOUGH TO CHANGE THE QUALITIES OF FOOD WITH MY THOUGHTS.

The second level of consciousness is the metaphysical level. The metaphysician understands that they can change the information of food, thereby changing what it does to and in the human body. I have used this technique with vegetarians who have been suffering from low iron to give their food more iron, and they have subsequently gone for blood tests and found their iron has gone up. It has worked every time!

The metaphysician uses the law of the universe that states, *"I can alter physical matter through my thoughts and intentions."* They understand their inherent mind power. I guess that's what this whole book has been about, so I will use this day to reinforce this to myself.

Angel Belief

I CAN TRANSFORM THE QUALITIES OF ANY FOOD JUST WITH MY THOUGHTS. IN FACT, I NOW RECOGNIZE I CAN TRANSFORM ANYTHING USING MY THOUGHTS AND INTENT.

From Elephant to Angel Action

With every single thing you eat today, before eating it, state the following in your mind or out loud if you are able to:

"I transform this food to be healthy, full of the highest nutrition, and full of life-giving energy. After eating it, all excess energy is released from my body. My body is whole and healthy and well, and is at its perfect weight easily and effortlessly. I look great in all of my clothes, and feel great too!"

DAY 81

Elephant Belief

ALL FOOD IS NOT EQUAL OR POSITIVE UNTIL I TRANSFORM IT TO BE SO.

The third level of consciousness is the mystical level. At the mystical level of thinking we understand that the Divine operates through us and through all things, and therefore all food is divine food, and full of divine love—all food!

At this level I do not have to do anything to transform the food, like I need to do at the metaphysical level of thinking.

At this level of thinking I am at an advanced level, as I understand the true nature of all food as inherently perfect and unable to do anything to harm me.

This is a giant leap in thinking and it begins in me today. Today I am not going to do anything to change the food I eat into either neutral or positive. Today I am going to really challenge my thinking so that I begin to see food as inherently neutral energy and positive energy ALREADY.

Food, other people, the environment—all are neutral energy and should be seen so! In fact they are positive energy only and always without requiring me to consciously change them at all.

Angel Belief

ALL FOOD IS INHERENTLY GOOD.

From Elephant to Angel Action

Each time you eat today think or say, *"This food is already perfect and life-giving right now. I can eat it knowing that it knows how to release itself from my body. I do not have to consciously do a thing!"*

NOW I AM A MASTER AND SO ARE YOU

Having completed this journey together, we are both at the fourth and final level of understanding ourselves, our bodies, and food. We are at the master level. This is the level where we understand that we are all One. We are all Whole. We are all Divine. No separation exists between the Divine Being within us and food, between the Divine Being and our bodies, and between the Divine Being and us.

Knowing this is a wonderful beginning, but as one cycle ends another begins, and as you complete this journey, you are now embarking on living this knowing each and every day of your life.

Having finished my own eighty-one days, I felt as though there was something huge and central that I had missed. I realized that the last part I needed to explore, that last lingering belief I needed to become aware of, was this:

I am trying to meet somebody else's idea of who I should be.

Why is this belief so central to everything I have already written about and everything I have already learned? The reason is because I may have undertaken this whole process successfully, but if I am still trying to be what other people expect me to be, I have essentially failed. The only reason I lie to myself, try too hard, get overwhelmed and stressed, worry and ignore my inner wisdom is because I am often trying to be what I think other people want me to be.

As I mentioned in earlier chapters, I am basing the sort of body I want to create on cultural and social norms. I am trying to become what the society of the day believes is successful and attractive. In this process I have essentially lost myself.

So, as I finish this part of my journey, I will free myself once and for all from doing this process or any other in order to meet somebody else's idea of who I should be. I can only be myself. I can only ever be myself in the here and now.

Why did I look at this belief at the end of the book rather than before I even began the journey? Because now I am ready to let it go. If I had challenged myself with this belief at the beginning, it would have overwhelmed me. And it would have overwhelmed you too! Now, together, we are ready to release the need to be anything other than who we already are.

A very close and talented friend of mine reminded me recently that there is no such thing as *loss* in the universe, only *release*. Applied to weight loss, you never needed to lose weight or lose anything. You have undertaken this whole journey to *release* old ways of being and thinking so that you can be transformed, and now you are just that.

As the MASTER that you now are, close your eyes for the last time on this journey and state to yourself, *"I have been living my life up until now trying to meet somebody else's idea of who I should be."*

Say this three times. Take a deep breath and imagine taking a special magic eraser and erasing this sentence as though it no longer exists. Rub it out as though by magic, so you cannot ever find it again.

Then state three times, *"I am living my own idea of who I am, and all I am is me. I am perfect just as I am."*

Congratulations. Today is the first day of the rest of your life. Go live it to the fullest, and enjoy all that you eat and all that you are, and do so knowing you are divine in every way! Thank you for walking this journey with me. Now it is time to walk your own journey. I walk beside you, just as you walked beside me.

With greatest love to you,

Helen Paige

REFERENCES

Beerlandt, Christiane. 2003. *The Key to Self-Liberation: 1000 Diseases and their Psychological Origins.* Eighth Edition. Beerlandt Publications.

Braden, Gregg. 2007. *The Divine Matrix: Bridging Time, Space, Miracles and Belief.* First Edition. Hay House Inc.

Grogan, Sarah. 2008. *Body Image: Understanding body dissatisfaction in men, women, and children.* Second Edition. Psychology Press.

Emoto, Masaru. 2001. *The Hidden Messages in Water.* Atria Books.

Hendricks, Gay. 2007. *Five Wishes: How answering one simple question can make your dreams come true.* Penguin Books.

Johnston, Anita. 2000. *Eating in the Light of the Moon: How women can transform their relationship with food through myths, metaphors and storytelling.* Gurze Books.

Lin, Chunyi. 2010. *Spring Forest Qigong Level One Manual.* Chunyi Lin.

Lipton, Bruce H. 2009. *The Biology of Belief: Unleashing the power of consciousness, matter and miracles.* Seventh Edition. Hay House Inc.

Newberg, Andrew, &. Waldman, Mark Robert. 2010. *How God Changes Your Brain: Breakthrough Findings from a Leading Neuroscientist.* Ballantine Books.

Pert, Candace B. 1997. *Molecules of Emotion: Why you feel the way you feel.* Simon & Schuster.

Ponder, Catherine. 1985. *The Healing Secrets of the Ages.* DeVorss & Co.

Rosas, Debbie. Rosas, Carlos. 2004. *The Nia Technique: The high powered energizing workout that gives you a new body and a new life.* Broadway Books.

Roth, Geneen. 2010. *Women Food and God.* Scribner.

Tate, Susan. 2011. *Wellness Wisdom: 31 ways to nourish your mind, body and spirit.* iUniverse.

ABOUT THE AUTHOR

Helen Paige is an author and teacher dedicated to raising the consciousness of the planet. Her dedication to living with authenticity, honesty, integrity and love shines through in all she is and does.

Born with her unique way of intuiting, Helen is able to see, feel and know where illness lies in the body as well as how to help the body to correct itself. She is an avid believer in the body's innate ability to heal itself, through releasing old patterns of beliefs, thoughts and emotions. She has spent the last 20 years working as a Medical Intuitive, helping many to gain insight into their illnesses and lives and inspiring people to live with renewed vitality and wholeness.

For more information on courses and other products by Helen please visit

www.HelenPaige.com

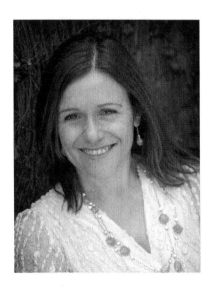

88327287R00141

Made in the USA
Middletown, DE
08 September 2018